MENDING MIRACLES

*Partnering With God
to Heal a Grieving Heart*

PAM VREDEVELT

Mending Miracles
Copyright © 2025 by Pam Vredevelt. All rights reserved.

No part of this book may be used or reproduced in any manner whatsoever without written permission, except in the case of brief quotations embodied in critical articles and reviews.

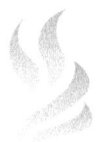

LIGHT SOURCE BOOKS

Published by Light Source

Printed in the United States of America.
ISBN-13: 978-0-9976876-2-0

WHAT PEOPLE ARE SAYING ABOUT MENDING MIRACLES

Pam Vredevelt writes with refreshing honesty and deep relatability. In Mending Miracles, her personal journey and the powerful stories she shares—paired with practical, faith-filled steps—offer a clear path to emotional healing and a deeper connection with God. This book is a lifeline for the hurting heart and a trusted companion for anyone seeking lasting wholeness.

Mary Kruse, *Lay Director Walk to Emmaus Texas*

In this profound work, Pam Vredevelt doesn't merely offer counsel—she extends an invitation to encounter the heart of God in the midst of our deepest pain. Drawing from decades of therapeutic experience and the raw grief of losing her son, she weaves together the wisdom of neuroscience, Scripture, and personal narrative to illuminate a path of healing. This book is not just a guide; it's a sacred journey toward restoration, where the Spirit meets us in our brokenness and leads us into wholeness.

Pam's authenticity and vulnerability create a space where readers can confront their own grief and find solace in the presence of a loving God. Her insights challenge us to move beyond mere survival and step into the fullness of life that God intends for us.

This is a must-read for anyone seeking healing after loss, offering not just hope, but a tangible pathway to emotional and spiritual renewal. In a world that often rushes past pain, Pam calls us to slow down, to grieve well, and to trust in the redemptive power of God's love. Mending Miracles is a resplendent North Star for those navigating the stormy seas of grief, offering guidance, comfort and courage to face the journey ahead.

Jamie Winship, *founder of Identity Exchange; best-selling author of Living Fearless: Exchanging the Lies of the World for the Liberating Truth of God*

In this groundbreaking book, Pam guides you on an intimate journey through the tumultuous shadows of grief, illuminating a Spirit-led path to wholeness. With unflinching honesty, she intertwines stories from forty years as a therapist, and the devastating loss of her sixteen-year-old son, with life-changing insights gleaned from brain science research, Biblical wisdom, and world thought leaders. This transformative work is not merely a guide but a rallying cry for connection and hope. It paves the way for personal encounters with God where you come to know that redeeming Love is always within reach, eager to mend your broken heart.

John Van Deist, *retired associate publisher, Tyndale; founder Multnomah Publishers, best-selling author*

When grief comes into our lives, we may or may not find a friend to walk with us. How can we expect others to enter into the strange and difficult pathways on which we find ourselves? True friends who come alongside and actually understand our heartache are rare and valuable. Pam Vredevelt is that sort of friend.

Mostly, I just want to say, "Wow!" Pam's writing is so warm, colorful, insightful, wise, and brimming over with feeling. She never, ever holds the reader at arm's length. Once we accept her invitation to enter the transformation experience she offers, we're swept along by truth and wonder—perhaps to healing places we never imagined going. Pam has walked the shadowed paths of sorrow, where heartache lingers. This is where she encountered the tender hand of God—mending what was broken, rekindling hope, and offering glimpses of heaven's love. Whether you are grieving now or simply seeking a deeper connection with God, Mending Miracles is a sacred invitation into God's healing presence - a gentle guide toward comfort, clarity, and quiet miracles of renewal.

> **Larry Libby,** *retired senior editor Multnomah Publisher/Penguin Random House; best-selling author of twenty-five books including* Someday Heaven, Who Made God?, *and* Angels, Angels Everywhere.

Each of us faces loss—whether it's the death of a loved one, a broken relationship, a lost dream, or a life-altering change. But navigating through grief in a way that leads to true, long-lasting healing? That is a rare gift. Pam Vredevelt, a seasoned professional counselor with a God-given gift for restoration, brings unparalleled wisdom and grace to the healing journey. In this powerful book, she serves as a compassionate guide, gently but firmly helping you stitch together the broken pieces of your heart.

With the precision of a skilled surgeon, she doesn't just help you manage grief; she shows you how to mend and heal in a deep, intimate partnership with God. In a world that too often silences the soul's wounds, Pam encourages us to tend to our emotional and spiritual well-being with the same care and intentionality we apply to our physical health.

Pam is one of the most Spirit-led healers of our time—her insight, wisdom, and love will transform your grief experience. If you've ever faced heartache or know someone who has, this book is essential reading. *Everyone* you know needs it. It is not just a book—it's a blueprint for restoration, and flourishing. Don't wait. Take a step toward the emotional freedom and wholeness you've been longing for.

> **Jenny Donnelly,** *Founder of Her Voice Movement*

Mending Miracles is more than just a book—it's a trusted guide for anyone walking through loss and grief. In these pages, Pam warmly invites readers to connect with the rhythm of God's heart—a heart that beats relentlessly for redemption and restoration. Drawing from the wisdom of Scripture and her own personal and professional experience, she shares powerful truths that reveal a God who not only leads you to victory but stays close to you in your pain. In this transformative journey, we learn how to draw closer to God -- whether our hearts are lifted in joyful celebration or aching with grief over life's painful contradictions.

I am filled with anticipation for the Kingdom impact this book will have—not only in our church but throughout our entire community. I believe healing is coming.

    Bret Williams, *Lead Pastor, Fireworks Church, San Antonio, Texas*

Pam's heartfelt storytelling and courageous honesty create a profound connection with the reader, inviting us into her agonies of grief and intimate encounters with God. Through raw and relatable stories, she opens a pathway for each of us to experience God as our companion in healing. Her ability to articulate the struggles we face while offering practical guidance equips us to navigate not only our deepest hurts but also the everyday challenges that leave us questioning, "What's next?" This book is a lifeline for anyone seeking hope, healing, and a life-giving relationship with God. A must-read for those yearning for greater clarity and freedom after any kind of disappointing loss.

    Debbie Woods, *Pharmacist*

If you've ever walked through the darkness of grief—or walked beside someone who has—you know how isolating and overwhelming it can feel. But what if healing didn't have to be as painful and lonely as it often seems? What if you had a wise friend to help light the way, offering *real* tools and grace for healing?

Mending Miracles is a must-read for anyone seeking emotional wholeness, or supporting others in a painful transition. Don't miss this. Experience the healing power of redeeming love and share it with friends in need.

Hannah Donnelly, *Singer, song-writer @hannahjewelmusic*

With heart-felt compassion, Pam's book leads you to reach inward and unlock your soul so that you can receive God's healing love. Her powerfully thought-provoking and moving book brings chills, tears, and joy. Pam writes both from the heart and from forty years of personal and clinical experience, revealing God's unconditional love in a quest to help you live life to your full potential.

Dr. Anita Myers, *Award-winning Restoration Dentist*

I love this book and plan to share it with many people. *Mending Miracles* helped me understand the lasting harm of unprocessed grief and how God can heal it. Pam combines deep personal insight, scientific clarity, and years of experience to offer practical steps toward emotional wholeness. After suffering several significant losses, I no longer feel emotionally flat—joy is now a daily part of my life. I highly recommend reading this book and doing the inner work. What do you have to lose?

Donna Chaney, *Appreciative Recipient*

Mending Miracles is life changing! Grief is a difficult and deeply personal journey—but through her transformative 'Love Talks' model, Pam demonstrates a deeply moving connection with God that invites you to personally experience God and receive whatever you need. Her integrative approach is rooted in faith, Scripture, and powerful scientific insight that speaks to the whole person—body, soul, and spirit. Love Talks will catalyze transformation in the deepest parts of who you are. If you're struggling, or just longing for more, *Mending Miracles* will meet you where you are and lovingly guide you toward greater peace and purpose.

Karen Bressel, *Woman of faith*

Mending Miracles is for anyone who has experienced any kind of loss. In her honest, open and vulnerable style, Pam shows us that no matter how subtle or great our loss may be, when we partner with God, He can help us transform our pain, confusion and loneliness into understanding, beauty and friendship with Him. In this life-changing book, Pam moves beyond offering encouragement and advice. She gives practical steps and teaches us how to breathe life into hope, to tell our story, to discover the Lord's nearness, to hear God, and to find truth that releases healing, purpose and peace. Thank you, Pam, for sharing your story and your gifts.

Reagan Miller, *Founder of Finding Virtue, a movement helping men raise sons to live God's truth in action*

Dedication

Although I've pondered the themes in this book for more than forty years, Mending Miracles was written over the course of two—years marked by a major cross-country move and profound life change. It is not the work of an academic or theologian, but the outpouring of a deeply personal journey. These pages flow from the lived experience of a wife, mother, researcher, professional counselor—and fellow traveler—seeking God in the midst of everyday demands, seasons of joy, and valleys of trauma and loss.

My hope is that Mending Miracles will draw you one step closer to real, soul-healing encounters with the living God—who promises to meet you in your pain, redeem what has been broken, and restore what has been lost.

This book is dedicated to you, and to all fellow travelers on the road toward hope and wholeness.

TABLE OF CONTENTS

Prologue: The Dream xiii
Chapter 1: We're in This Together 1
Chapter 2: Making Space to Mend 11
Chapter 3: Your Story Matters 21
Chapter 4: Where Healing Happens Best 45
Chapter 5: Reset 57
Chapter 6: The Power of Truth 67
Chapter 7: What's the Bigger Picture? 73
Chapter 8: The Secret of Surrender 79
Chapter 9: Recognize with Compassion 89
Chapter 10: Angel Visits in the Dark 101
Chapter 11: God Encounters 113
Chapter 12: Tear Tracking 121
Chapter 13: Love Talks 127
Chapter 14: Hearing Matters 135
Chapter 15: Release and Receive 147
Chapter 16: Grace Gifts 159
Chapter 17: Eternal Dreams 175
Chapter 18: Mystery on Heaven's Doorstep 181
Chapter 19: Chocolate Chip Cookies? 187
Chapter 20: There's No Place Like Home 203
Chapter 21: Redeeming Loss 223
Acknowledgements..283

PROLOGUE

THE DREAM

I gasped in astonishment, bolting upright in bed, fixated on his last words: *Redeeming loss.* Mystery hung heavy in the midnight air. Rubbing my eyes, I wondered if something eternally significant was happening.

Brain science says you and I average three to five dreams a night. Most of mine end in oblivion, but not this one. This dream—a full-body technicolor experience unlike any other I had experienced—nagged at me for weeks.

While fast asleep, I was wide awake in another realm, flying on a jumbo jet to meet with John Vandiest, chief operating officer of a publishing house. Decades had passed since I signed my first book contract with his company for *Empty Arms: Hope and Emotional Support for Those Who Have Suffered a Miscarriage, Stillbirth, or Tubal Pregnancy.*

Somewhere beyond time and space and my conscious awareness, the dream unfolded like I was watching a film at a local theater.

> I'm wheeling a suitcase out of a large hotel lobby, and down a hallway toward my room.
>
> I hear a latch click and a door opens on my right. Much to my surprise, Hannah Donnelly walks into the hall.[1] Laughing out loud I throw open my arms, wrap her in a big bear hug, and say, "Hannah Donnelly! What are you doing here?!"
>
> Sporting a sunny smile she says, "I'm going to the meeting!"
>
> We exchange a few words and agree to catch up later. I continue down the tidal green, smokey blue Lithuanian carpet toward my room.
>
> Just ahead, a door clunks closed, startling me from pleasant thoughts of warm cookies in the lobby. Amy Grant steps into the hall on my right.[2]
>
> Delightfully surprised, we happily hug, and I say, "Amy Grant! It's so good to see you! What are you doing here?"
>
> In Amy's gentle style, she smiles warmly and says, "I'm going to the meeting!"
>
> The three of us are unaware of the agenda. We simply know it's imperative to show up.
>
> When the time comes, we enter a large room together, surrounded by floor-to-ceiling mirrors. The meeting venue reminds me of a large ballet or exercise studio, yet different. The dark brown wood floorboards look more like those of an old well-worn theater stage than a fine polished dance surface.

I see the chief publisher standing on the far side of the room, holding several large books in his arms. Eager to connect, I walk in his direction, Hannah and Amy following close behind.

We greet each other like good friends who haven't seen each other in years. Bursting with curiosity, I can't stop myself from asking, "John, what are we doing here?"

Handing a book to each of us he says, "I invited you here to read from a screenplay."

Having no frame of reference for this sort of thing, I wonder how I can contribute something of value that is worth his time. In an effort to relieve my angst, I ask, "What is the screenplay about?"

John tilts his head left, looks at me like he's hiding a secret, and replies, "Redeeming loss."

For God speaks again and again, though people do not recognize it. He speaks in dreams, in visions of the night, when deep sleep falls on people as they lie on their beds.[3]

Rewind 40 Years Ago

I recall encountering a similar mystery after our first baby died halfway to term. I walked into my five-month check-up wearing a colorful maternity dress, excited to hear our baby's heartbeat. Instead, I heard the doctor say, "I'm not picking up a heartbeat, Pam. There doesn't appear to be any fetal movement. I think the baby is dead. I don't know why but we will know more after labor and delivery."

Forty-eight hours later, my husband, John, and I left the hospital with broken hearts and empty arms.

A young couple, we were completely unprepared for the emotional devastation.

The more you love, the more you hurt.

The deeper the bond, the deeper the pain.

We began the long dark road of grief asking the same questions you might ask: *What do we do? Where do we start? How do we pick up the pieces and mend our shattered hearts?*

A few weeks later, I resumed swimming laps at our athletic club, crying my way back and forth across the pool. God got an earful that day: *God, we prayed every day for our baby! Why didn't you answer? How can anything good come from this? What's the point? Are you even there? God, I need perspective!*

At the end of my emotional spew, much to my surprise, the image of a book appeared in my mind. Instantly I knew it was a book for broken-hearted moms and dads grieving the loss of their baby. Though it didn't fully make sense, something about that image was setting the stage for a larger purpose.

I'd never written a book and knew nothing about the process.

Was I being invited to write? I didn't know. Frankly, the idea seemed daunting.

The following day, I called a mentor-friend who was a published writer and told her about my experience in the pool. Without hesitation she said, *I want to see the first three chapters of your story by Monday.* It was Friday.

Her insistence rubbed me wrong. I snapped back, *There's no way. I'm not ready for that!*

She chose words carefully, cloaking truth with compassion: *Pam, you have to do this now and capitalize on your current experience. Your perspective will change over time.*

Though I didn't want to admit it, the truth resonated with me.

Reluctantly, I started spilling my story onto a yellow-lined pad of paper the next day. The longer I wrote, the more my pen picked up speed across the page. I didn't know if I could write well, or if what I wrote would matter to anyone else. I simply followed what I perceived as a divine prompt.

A few months later I sent three chapters and a book outline to several different publishing houses. Some never responded. But, much to my astonishment, representatives from three companies wanted to meet with me to discuss a contract. I ended up signing with Multnomah/Penguin Random House because it seemed like the best fit for me.

The following year, *Empty Arms* was published. Liz Haney, my editor, walked into my hospital room on June 13th where I joyfully cradled our newborn daughter, Jessie. Handing me my first copy of the book hot off the press, she smiled and said, "No more empty arms!"

Shortly after we brought Jessie home, Liz called to say that *Empty Arms* was a Golden Medallion Book Award finalist. I didn't know what that meant, but she seemed over-the-moon thrilled. I guessed it meant that someone, somewhere, thought my writing had value. In all honesty, Liz is brilliantly gifted. She took what I sent to her and turned water into wine. To this day, that little book continues to offer hope and healing to hurting moms and dads around the world.

After the Dream

Replays of John Vandiest handing Hannah, Amy, and me the screenplay continued to nag at me. Was God saying something to me in the dream? If so, what was the message?

In the past, I might have chalked up the dream to too much pizza. Not anymore. I'm better at listening and paying attention to God than I was three decades ago. I've also learned to ask God questions and to watch for answers that come in whispers, nudges, dreams, and pictures. God's love language is highly creative and customized for each individual.

I pay attention because I simply don't want to miss anything God might ask me to partner in for the greater good. Why talk yourself out of something God may be inviting you into? It's much more fun to explore possibilities.

Many years had passed since John Vandiest and I last talked. He was at least twenty years ahead of me. Not knowing if he was still alive or where he lived, I reached out to his son-in-law, Don Jacobson, who is also a prominent leader in the publishing world.

Don was kind enough to pass along John's personal phone number. Within an hour, John and I enjoyed a happy reunion, updating one another on family and other important matters.

It took a while, but I finally worked up the courage to explain the reason for my call. Honestly, I felt a bit awkward. It isn't common practice for me to spontaneously dial an industry leader and discuss a personal dream. Not everyone is comfortable talking about subjects like this.

Clumsily finding my way, I began: *John, you may leave this call as puzzled as I am, but I recently had a vivid dream, and you were in it. I sense there may be something significant about it, but I'm not certain. I'm wondering if I can describe the dream for you and if you might share your thoughts with me?*

John was most gracious and listened attentively to the details. Genuinely interested, he peppered our conversation with questions and suggested I contact specific individuals.

After our conversation, I pressed pause to take time to pray and reflect.

After living in the Pacific Northwest for over forty years, our family was in the middle of a major life transition. Our adult children and grandchildren surprised us one evening with curious news. They said they believed God was leading them to move to the Texas hill country and they didn't want to go without us. They asked us to pray about going with them.

To make a long story short, within one short week, John and I separately knew the Lord was nudging us to go. The specifics were not yet defined about where we'd land in Texas, but we agreed to move with the family. Over the next few months, we packed our belongings, sold our homes, and sought God's guidance.

Similar to my experience after the loss of our baby, the idea of a writing project seemed daunting in the midst of such huge changes. But I couldn't shake the dream or echoes of the whisper: *redeeming loss*. Peace came in knowing that when God initiates a plan, He orchestrates ways to see things through, often via agencies we can't possibly anticipate. I simply needed to pay attention, trust, and follow His lead.

Cliff Notes—Seeking God for Wisdom

I sensed a nudge to call my friend, Cindy,[4] a creative leader gifted with discernment. I was curious to know how she perceived the dream. She listened and shared intuitive perspectives as I took copious notes. These writings combined with those in my prayer notebook emerged into a brief summary of meanings:

- **Hannah and Amy**— These women are vocal artists representing two generations and distinct markets, sharing their talents across both faith-based and mainstream platforms.

- **Singers** -- are musical story tellers that use their voices to weave memory, stir emotion, and carry listeners into experience. Their songs are both a map and message, guiding hearts and minds alike.

- **A timely message is needed by multiple generations across diverse groups.**

- **Airplane**—symbolic of traveling to new heights in spiritual awareness, discernment, and influence.

- **Hotel Hallway**— A hallway is a transitional space, symbolizing the movement from one phase of life to the next. It's a place of connection—linking past to future, one room to the next, and people to new experiences. It can stir mixed emotions—excitement, vulnerability, and apprehension—as transition represents both the uncertainty and the potential of what lies ahead.

- Hallway on the **left**—symbolic of things you receive

- Doors on the **right**—symbolic of opportunity[5], access to God[6], something you walk through and have faith to release and give away [7].

- **Three distinct rooms**—each symbolizing a unique mindset reached by different modes of engagement.

- **Screenplay**—A medium that brings a story to life, allowing audiences to see, hear, and experience its message. It outlines scenes, provides dialogue, and offers detailed guidance for character interactions, making the narrative both vivid and accessible.

- **Reader of a Screenplay**—One who steps into the role of a character, bringing a story to life. The reader interprets the written word and creatively imitates[8] a character in ways that best engage the full range of human senses for maximum impact.

- **Well-Worn Stage**—A platform marked by time and use, where a message refined through practice takes on new life with each telling. Like a well-worn glove or a favorite pair of shoes, the message fits with ease—shaped by experience and made powerful through transformation, both in the one who delivers it and those who receive it.

- **A stage is set to display God's redeeming love.**
- **Dance studio**—a dedicated space for learning and practicing dance with music and movement, offering a safe and supportive environment where individuals of all ages and skill levels can grow through hands-on experiential training.
- **Mirrors**—The meeting room was lined with floor-to-ceiling mirrors, symbolizing God's presence where the Spirit of Truth reveals ultimate reality.[9] Mirrors reflect images,[10] enabling us to see things as they truly are—and ourselves as we truly are. In every human being, mirrors echo the reflection of God's image, reminding us of our divine connection.

Walking our Property with God

I had a conversation with God today while walking the property. Much of what we've known for forty years is stripped away. We are living in an RV on-site while building a multi-generational home with our adult kids and grandchildren.

In the midst of these disruptive changes, I need perspective. A shortened version of my conversation follows. What I sense God say to me is italicized.

> God, who do you say that I am in this new place and new season of life?
>
> *You are perfume; a Kingdom culture shifter.*[11]
>
> I believe you were speaking to me in the dream. What do you want me to do?

> *I want you to guide and guard the broken-hearted. Equip those I love to partner with Me and mend their wounds, so they can flourish and fulfill their purposes.*
>
> *You must RISK. Move beyond your comfort zone. Trust Me with outcomes. Offer language, pictures, and truth that demonstrate how to see, hear, and partner with Me. Tell your miracle and mystery stories. Share our talks and what you know. You have everything you need.*

Your encouragement to *risk* reminds me of wise words that I recorded a while back in my journal:

> There are two fearsome journeys any serious believer must take in order to fully flourish and love as You (God) loved: The first is the journey to hidden vulnerability (the willingness to bear burdens and expose ourselves to risks that no one else can fully see or understand.) The second is sacrifice (the choice to voluntarily choose to turn toward the pain and loss in our world and in our own heart, like Jesus did, in order to redeem it.)[12]

A golden thread weaves through what You are saying to me now, and these words. Today I say "Yes," and accept your invitation. I commit my time, energy, and gifts to You for this special purpose. Please clarify the risks you want me to take, and give me the courage to take them.

I trust you to provide the language and stories that will achieve the outcomes you desire. I trust you to multiply what is offered for the greater good of each person you love and call by name.

Thank you for inviting me into this adventure. I look to you to orchestrate the way. Though I don't know where you are taking us, I believe it will be good.

Breathe. Inhale deeply. Slowly exhale.

Ready by faith, here we go...

Two Years Later

The book you now hold in your hands is the result of seeking God for meaning in an unexpected dream—and accepting His invitation to write again. Each chapter was born in solitude, and shaped over hours and months at a small tray table in our RV. It was there, in stillness and surrender, that the message slowly took form.

These pages hold reflections of a forty-year journey—my own, in company with many others who also longed for truth, hope, and healing. I invite you to come with me, to see what unfolded, and to listen for what God might whisper to your heart, too. As you read, my earnest prayer is that you feel less alone—and that, along the way, you experience the same comfort, clarity, and healing peace that kept finding me as I wrote the following pages for you.

It's not where your dreams take you, it's where you take your dreams.
Maya Angelou

1

WE'RE IN THIS TOGETHER

God, where were you? I was there, my child.
I was the peace. I was the breath. I was the comfort.
Lindsey O'Connor

Hello. Welcome to a safe place.

I'm guessing you picked up this book because you are hurting, or someone you love needs more support. I want to assure you that you are not alone. Each one of us grieves deeply and recurrently throughout life. Your grief is as unique as your fingerprint.

Great sorrow, as you know, can pull you into a black vortex that feels virtually inescapable.

Perhaps that's why you are here. You're not yourself. You can't focus. You're running on fumes. Your friends and loved ones need you. You want to feel better, but you're not sure how to get there. The path of healing is elusive. Yet, something deep inside you says, *It's time.*

It's time to stop sinking into the dark abyss and begin moving toward the light again. It's time to stop expecting yourself to carry this heavy grief alone. It's time to stop searching within for all the answers. It's time to start living as you were designed—to move through grief in friendship with God. Will you give yourself permission to explore ways to share the weighty burdens that have been draining the life from you?

My name is Pam, and it is my honor and privilege to help you find the path forward toward wholeness where you can flourish in your God-given purpose. Your well-being matters, especially to God and those who love you most. I want to offer what I can to help.

In the pages ahead, I hope to pass along some of what I've learned during four decades as a licensed professional counselor, and as a fellow traveler through dark valleys. I've been blessed to have been trained by incredible giants in the fields of trauma therapy, neuropsychiatry, and grief (Bessel van der Kolk, Dan Siegel, Norm Wright, Warner Swarner, and David Kessler to name a few). I'm deeply grateful for all they've taught me.

As much as I've gained from these remarkable pioneers, the most exceptional teachers I've learned from and alongside are God, my family, spiritual mentors, and the people I've served in the counseling office over four decades. You'll notice their shaping influences on me in the pages ahead.

I'm wondering if your family openly discussed how to deal with loss and grief when you were growing up. Most people I talk to, did not. I didn't either. And four years of graduate school didn't offer me many clues.

There are good reasons why most of us don't know what to say, and often feel powerless to help people who are hurting, including ourselves. With little awareness or tools, it's no wonder we find ourselves overwhelmed and powerless against the fierce force of grief. Perhaps you worry, like I once did, that if you let yourself feel your feelings (sadness, fear, anger, guilt, or regret), you'll end up drowning in them. Or if you talk about your grief, people will feel awkward and go away, leaving you even more sad and lonely than before. Perhaps silence feels safer.

These are common struggles and ones that I wrestled with, too, after our first baby suddenly died halfway to term. My heart was cracked wide open. I didn't know where to start or what to do. Conflicting thoughts and emotions raced in and out with no logical progression.

Seriously, there were moments when I secretly wondered if I was losing my mind.

As a young twenty-something, I was well aware that I resisted and blocked my feelings. It seemed *easier*, or at least more *manageable* to ignore the grief, stuff it, and hold it at bay by keeping busy.

The problem is, *avoidance isn't healthy. It's self-abandonment.*

When we ignore painful feelings, we end up forsaking a very important part of who we are, and how God designed us. Counselors have a fancy name for these addictive efforts to escape reality. They're called maladaptive coping mechanisms and they don't work. Scientific research says they cause more harm than good.

Obviously, there is a time and place for setting aside or tuning out painful feelings. We need to be able to emotionally unplug from grief so that we can be present with our family and friends, attend to our work, and manage daily responsibilities.

But putting your heart on hold indefinitely will rob you of vitality, freedom, and quality of life.

The truth is: *What you resist, persists.*

Fast forward to after the loss of our first baby. Our daughter, Jessie, was born two years later, on the same day my book, *Empty Arms*, arrived hot off the press. Jessie burst into this world full of energy, alert, bright-eyed, and attentively watching everything going on around her. Three years later our son, Benjamin, arrived. Cradling our solid, strong, close-to-ten-pound baby, we soon recognized his innate sensitivity to people and music. Wonderfully satisfied being a family of us four and no more, we decided we were "done having children."

Then, out of the blue, I turned up pregnant. How could it be? Well, I knew how it *could* be, but it shouldn't have been! We'd taken all the precautions. Somehow, this baby was conceived in spite of the foolproof birth-control we'd used for seventeen years. I guess we didn't have as much control as I thought.

Life has a knack for teaching us that "control" is really an illusion.

At the time, my emotions resembled a tossed salad: a wedge of guilt here, a slice or two of anger there, with some self-pity sprinkled over the top for spice. *Guilt*…because I had friends who wanted so very much to get pregnant and couldn't—and here I was upset that the little test stick had turned blue. *Anger*…because my agenda had been interrupted and rearranged. *Self-pity*…because I was sick all day every day through most of the pregnancy.

When I was three months pregnant, I was invited to speak at a major women's conference but couldn't help wondering why I was there given my inner turmoil.

Bottom line: I was annoyed because I didn't *want* to be sick or pregnant. One morning during the conference, I had some time off the platform, so I ordered breakfast in my room, read the Gospel of John, and wrote down my thoughts and feelings. I can assure you God got an earful.

But then, after I'd vented, it was *His* turn. There have been times through the years when God has made something very clear to me, and this was one of those times. While reading John 15, two familiar sentences suddenly hit me like a whopping dose of smelling salts.

Jesus was speaking: I am the true Vine, and My Father is the vinedresser. Every branch in Me that does not bear fruit, He takes away; and every *branch* that continues to bear fruit, He repeatedly prunes, so that it will bear more fruit even richer and finer fruit.[13]

What I sensed God saying to me was, "Pam, you're not being set back; you're being *pruned* back."

In that instant, a picture of the three rosebushes in our front yard came to mind. Each summer the bushes produce huge, long-stemmed yellow roses that fill our home with amazing fragrance. Arranged in a vase on a table, the blooms seem to glow with a golden light of their own.

But in the fall, John cuts them back. *Way* back. After his pruning shears are done, I look at those stumps and think, "My goodness, the man is ruthless. Those poor things look decapitated!" Every fall I wonder if they'll ever grow back and…sure enough, every spring they teem with life more vibrant than the year before.

Pam, you're not being set back; you're being pruned back.

In the stillness of God's presence, I knew He was up to something—and that my pregnancy had in no way caught Him by surprise. For some incomprehensible reason, a higher good was working to produce more beauty and fragrance in my life.

Little did I know that our precious little boy, Nathan, would arrive six weeks early, with a surprise diagnosis of Down syndrome and severe heart complications. I'll tell you more about Nathan later, but for now, I want to bring the focus to you and your story.

When you're dealing with an ending, particularly a change you didn't intentionally choose, it's hard work to figure out how to settle into a new normal. Transitions evoke intense, erratic, and difficult emotions.

We really don't want to swallow our feelings. Something inside warns us against burying our emotions alive, but it's often a struggle to not do so.

Does any of this sound familiar?

What makes healing our heart wounds so challenging?

Our natural instinct as human beings is to avoid pain and pursue pleasure. It's hard-wired into our body, to keep us alive. That's why it feels counter-intuitive to intentionally turn toward difficult emotions rather than avoid them.

I learned a long time ago that good intentions don't heal. Taking action does.

On the heels of my own losses, I knew I needed to take care of my broken heart. The counseling office had given me a front-row seat to witness the brutal devastation and generational impact of unresolved grief in far too many families.

Please grab ahold of this important truth and don't let go.

ature that isn't transformed, is transmitted.

Do you remember the lesson about heat, energy, and motion in high-school physics? The first law of thermodynamics? It says that energy cannot be created or destroyed, it can only be changed from one form to another. In other words, energy doesn't disappear or go away. It only gets moved around or used in different ways.

So, what does physics have to do with grief?

Grief is the intense physical and emotional distress we experience after any kind of loss or trauma.

Here's a simple way to think about emotion: *E-motion = Energy in motion.*

Grief is a fierce force of energy in motion that flows through your body. You can probably recall moments after your loss when you sensed more tension in your neck, chest, stomach, legs, arms, and core of your being.

Grieving a loss is a full-body experience. The imprint of loss remains in your being and your body keeps score.[14]

This is why it's critical to learn how to proactively treat emotional wounds with practices that harness and use grief energy for positive change.

When we neglect our heart wounds, not only do we harm ourselves, we also hurt those we love and care about the most. Invalidated, unresolved emotional pain that remains buried turns toxic and damages our health and relationships.[15] That's the bad news.

The point of this book is to share good news and to equip you with tools that empower emotional healing so that you can flourish in fulfilling your purpose. Here's where rays of hope begin to break through.

You are designed with an innate ability to partner with God and safe friends in healing your heart wounds to thrive. Mending a broken heart is not all up to you. It is not a do-it-yourself task.

And it's not all up to God. Passive resignation to, "There's nothing I can do," won't help you feel better or improve anything. You are neurologically designed to heal best in the context of loving relationships[16] and to actively participate *with* God in mending your heart so that you can fulfill specific purposes in this world. What do I mean?

Better yet, what might that look like?

"We're called to a very specific kind of work," writes John Mark Comer, "to make a Garden-like world where image bearers can flourish and thrive, where people can experience and enjoy God's generous love. A kingdom where God's will is done 'on earth as it is in heaven,' where the glass wall between earth and heaven is so thin and clear and translucent that you don't even remember it's there. That's the kind of world we're called to make. After all, we're just supposed to continue what God started in the beginning."[17]

Andy Crouch, another creative thought leader, offers an additional perspective:

> "What are we meant to be? We are meant to flourish. Not just to survive but to thrive; not just to exist but to explore and expand…To flourish is to be fully alive, and when we read or hear those words something about us wakes up, sits up a bit straighter, and leans ever so slightly forward. To be fully alive would not just connect us to our own proper human purpose, but also to the very heights and depths of divine glory. To live fully in these transitory lives on this fragile earth, in such a way that we somehow partner with the glory of God—that would be flourishing. And that is what we are meant to do."[18]

Yes! Like the butterfly that flaps its wings and flies free from its entombing chrysalis, you are designed to experience transformation in dark desolate places and to emerge more fully alive and fully free.

You are far more valuable and resilient than you think.

When you partner with God in giving your broken heart the proper care and attention it needs, the emotional energy of grief becomes fuel for positive transformation. It may be hard to believe right now, but it really is possible for you to experience a new, vibrant increased capacity to love life and thrive.

As we begin, may I make a couple of requests regarding the time we spend together?

First, I ask that you bring something important with you. I call it the HOW of any growth adventure. In order to get every possible benefit from this experiential journey, please come to the pages ahead with an **H**onest, **O**pen, and **W**illing heart.

Now think carefully about how you want to answer the second request. The quality of your life and the well-being of the following generations are riding on your decision.

Are you willing to start taking your emotional pain as seriously as you take physical pain?

Or, in other words, *are you willing to start paying attention to your inner world as much as you pay attention to your outer world?*

Pause a moment. Read that section again, and really think about it.

If your answer happens to be, "No," that's okay. I trust you to know when you're ready.

One of the greatest gifts we've been given is the gift of choice. You always have choices, and I believe that you know yourself better than others. What's most important is that you don't put your heart on hold for long and that you make space to mend sooner rather than later.

You're worth the time and effort!

If you're ready, let's get started. I'm eager to meet you inside.

Now, breathe.

You're not alone.

An Invitation to Action

Consider making a decision to commit to the following choices:

1. I choose to be Honest, Open, and Willing during this transformation experience.

2. I make a commitment to myself to give my broken heart the proper care and attention it needs, and to respond to my emotional pain as I would to my physical aches and pain.

3. I will make time to partner with God and learn how to use the energy of grief for positive transformation and growth, rather than allowing it to steal my joy and ability to heal.

2

MAKING TIME TO MEND

He that lacks time to mourn, lacks time to mend.
Maya Angelou

All change involves loss.

After any loss—whether it's the loss of a loved one, a significant relationship, a job, a beloved pet, your health, home, friend group, or anything else that deeply matters to you, your world is temporarily thrown into chaos.

All that you've learned and know about life is wildly disrupted, shaken, and challenged. The neural maps in your brain, formed from your prior experiences, must be rewired from *what you were used to*, to your new reality *as it is* now.

Warning: The danger after a loss is to resist change by re-enacting past scripts, instead of writing a new screenplay for your story.

What might that look like?

I have fond memories of Sara, who came to see me because her medical doctor insisted. Her joy had been gone for years, replaced by a persistent gray mood. "It seems like I'm always sad and worried. I don't like it, but I don't know how to feel better," she explained.

During our time together, I learned about her history and the important life events she experienced. Like a TV newscaster reporting daily events, she mentioned that she gave birth to a stillborn daughter fourteen years ago. The following year, her mom died, and her son was born. Seven months after giving birth to their baby boy, her husband was transferred, and they moved clear across the country to make a new home in California.

Her voice was machine-like, flat, and void of emotion.

When I asked about her stillborn daughter, she said that it happened without warning. The doctor gave them the sad news; her husband couldn't bear it and promptly left the hospital.

She decided that night, alone in her little hospital room, to put the whole thing behind her and never talk about it. From that moment on, she blocked it, pushed it to the back of her mind, and with a single-minded focus, determined to get on with her life. It seemed like the best choice for everyone. She and her husband both grew up in families that lived by the "no talk" rule when it came to anything sad. She told me, "It doesn't do any good to dredge up the past. It just makes things worse, not better."

But here's the problem. *Resisting grief doesn't make it go away. It simply drives it underground.*

For fourteen years, Sara used huge amounts of energy to push away the grief related to the loss of her baby. As we talked about her daughter, all that buried emotion erupted like a giant geyser, every bit as intense and as real as if she had lost the baby yesterday.

Sara broke the "no talk" rule and made a fresh start toward healing. Even though she didn't know how long it would take and couldn't see very far ahead, she was **H**onest, **O**pen, and **W**illing. It was a life-changing new beginning.

> *I have learned now that while those who speak about one's miseries usually hurt, those who keep silent hurt more.*
>
> C. S. Lewis

Loss rips and tears our hearts. We are born to bond. When connections are severed by losses we didn't choose, and over which we have no control, inner bleeding occurs.

The greater the bond, the greater the pain.

Do you know what happens when you pull apart two pieces of paper, stuck together with superglue? You're left with a messy torn-up jumble of scrappy bits and pieces. It's a fitting picture of your heart after loss.

That's why it's critical to proactively take small, calculated steps to gather the shattered pieces of your heart and tend to them with as much care as you would a broken limb. If you were to break your arm, would you tell yourself to ignore the pain, keep busy, and take your mind off of it? I don't think so. You'd see a doctor as soon as possible because you want your arm to quickly heal without complications or any loss of function.

We usually don't ignore physical wounds because we know that if we do, other problems can arise and make matters worse. We promptly visit a doctor for a broken limb and trust them to realign bones, prevent infection, and prescribe whatever treatment is necessary. We follow their guidance to fully heal.

Emotional wounds are similar. They may be invisible to the naked eye, but they are no less real and no less influential in determining the quality of your life. Trying to shut out your feelings only turns your heartache into more of a tyrant. The pain becomes louder and more insistent, like a person pressing your doorbell, who won't stop until you open the door.

Most of us underestimate the significant impact of loss. We minimize our experience by saying, "It's not a big deal. Everyone goes through it." We simply didn't learn the facts along the way: Heartbreaking loss hits your brain like a Mack truck. Neuroscience has shown that a painful loss triggers the same mechanisms in your brain that are activated when addicts withdraw from cocaine or opioids.

When you're grieving, the typical instincts you ordinarily rely on can lead you in the wrong direction. *You cannot always trust your thoughts because grief distorts your perception.*

Clinical research shouts a clear warning: Do not run from grief!

Avoiding and suppressing painful emotions leads to increased negative ruminations, anxiety, depression, prolonged suffering, and complicated grief.[19] It seems to me that those in the health and wellness industry need to be sending a warning:

> *Avoiding grief is hazardous to your health and relationships.*

So, the pressing question is: What are you doing to take care of your heart? Are you automatically defaulting to messages you learned in the past such as: *Don't talk. Don't trust. Don't feel*, similar to Sara, or are you practicing proven strategies that promote healing?

Taking care of your grieving heart isn't a selfish act, or just a nice idea. It's a strategic choice for your physical, mental, and relational well-being.

I can promise you this: You'll never regret being intentional about making time to mend. The returns on your investment will serve you and those you love very well through the rest of your life. It's key to feeling better and finding peace and purpose.

> *The real voyage of discovery consists not in seeing new landscapes, but in having new eyes.*
>
> *Marcel Proust*

Record Your Progress—Write to Heal

Ignored grief is like trying to drive with a windshield smeared in thick mud and no way to clean it. It clouds your vision, distorts your perception, and makes it nearly impossible to move forward with clarity or confidence.

There is a better way. If you've come this far, I believe you have chosen to pay attention to what is often ignored and to take responsibility for your well-being. Emotional healing progresses slowly as you learn to pause, intentionally face your heartache with God's help, and bit by bit, release your grief.

Our minds are designed to try to understand the things that happen to us. When we suffer loss, we work overtime to make sense of the experience and find meaning. Writing allows us to pause, listen to our hearts, and intentionally focus on what matters.

We step back, pay attention, and sort through our experiences. By translating our loss into language and putting a pen to paper, we engage in healthy grief release.

James W. Pennebaker has shown in decades of research that "actively holding back or inhibiting our thoughts and feelings can be hard work. Over time, the work of inhibition gradually undermines the body's defenses. Like other stressors, inhibition can affect immune function, the action of the heart and vascular systems, and even the biochemical workings of the brain and nervous systems. Holding back thoughts and feelings places people at risk for both major and minor diseases."[20]

Opening up, on the other hand, has the opposite effect. Pennebaker says, "When disclosing deeply personal experiences, there are immediate changes in brainwave patterns, skin conductance levels, etc. after confessions. Significant drops in blood pressure and heart rate, as well as improvements in immune function occur. In the weeks and months after opening up, people's physical and psychological health is improved."[21]

Turns out that there is a lot of scientific evidence to support the therapeutic value of opening up and writing about our losses. Brain SPECT Imaging[22] shows us that the act of writing accesses the left brain, which is analytical and rational. While the left brain is occupied, the right brain is free to perceive, create, and feel. Writing clears the mind of mental blocks and helps us tap into added brainpower to creatively think through matters and sort things out.

People who write about their traumatic experiences report improved memory, less depression, more happiness, fewer trips to the doctor, and overall improved health. They also feel happier and less negative than before they began writing. Depressive symptoms, ruminations, and general anxiety tend to drop in the weeks and months after writing occurs.[23]

Multiple studies show that writing helps us come to terms with trauma and reduces its negative impact on our physical health.[24] It strengthens immune cells and can decrease symptoms of asthma and rheumatoid arthritis.[25] People suffering from Post-Traumatic Stress Disorder (PTSD) who write about their experiences report fewer flashbacks, nightmares, and intrusive painful memories. These improvements enable them to slowly re-engage in activities and places that they'd otherwise avoid.[26]

> **THE POSITIVE IMPACT OF FOCUSED WRITING**
>
> The effect of two types of journaling were compared during a one-month study.
>
> - One group wrote about their deep feelings related to a personal trauma.
> - A second group recorded their deep feelings and thoughts about their trauma.
> - A third group focused their writing on factually reporting events.
> - Results: Journaling about a personal trauma facilitated positive growth. However, the focus of journaling was important. Writing that expressed emotions and thoughts while trying to make sense of the trauma, with a focus on looking for the positive gifts inherent in suffering, showed significantly greater benefits than journaling focused strictly on the expression of painful emotion. Writers who focused on painful emotion alone reported more symptoms of illness during the study.[27]

Even writing for only twenty minutes a day can rewire the brain and facilitate healing.[28] As you write, you discover new insights, inspirations, and capacities that empower you to keep moving forward *through* the shadows.

You are more resilient than you may think.

> **ADVANTAGES OF JOURNALING**
>
> Those who practice journaling:
>
> - Are re-employed sooner after losing their jobs
> - Miss fewer days of work
> - Have higher grade point averages
> - Show better overall sporting performances
> - Have better working memories[29]

A small window of regular writing can also increase your insight and awareness of God. It positions you to receive fresh perspective, comfort, and renewal. It's easier to hear God whisper in quiet stillness.[30] As you pause and pay attention to your inner longings, you develop vital skills that fortify your resolve, nurture resilience, and equip you to reclaim joy.

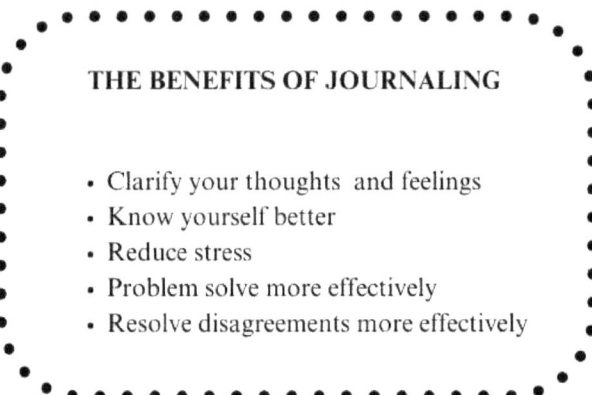

THE BENEFITS OF JOURNALING

- Clarify your thoughts and feelings
- Know yourself better
- Reduce stress
- Problem solve more effectively
- Resolve disagreements more effectively

As we continue exploring together, I invite you to write about your loss, at your own pace. Aim for small incremental steps. Please be gentle with yourself. This is not a time to push hard.

I'll supply you with a toolbox of healing strategies.[31] You get to choose when to pick up your pen and record your experiences.

If, at any time, your grief is too overwhelming, remind yourself that you are safe. Give yourself permission to take a break. Breathe deeply, ask God for help, and come back to writing when you have the energy to do so. Your grief is as unique as your fingerprint.

How you feel is how you feel. It's OK.

Keeping a written record is a personal way to honor the essence and meaning of your loss, and to keep track of your tangible progress. It can also become a reference point in the future when you face new and different losses and want to support others through their grief. When it comes to your written record, the choices are all yours.

I'm here to guide and guard you along the way. It's truly my honor to walk with you.

An Invitation to Action

1. Choose a notebook solely for recording your healing progress. You'll use it for a while, so select something attractive that you like with lined or blank pages. It will be your private place to capture thoughts, feelings, and insights that emerge in your transformation experience.

2. Select a 15–30-minute time slot, four times a week, and mark these on your calendar. Protect this time to the best of your ability. Choose a time of day when your energy is typically better than others and when it's easier to be consistent. Consider keeping a small bag with your journal, pens, markers, and whatever else you want, so that it's easy to transport if you need to shift your plan. You'd be surprised how many moms and executives do good transformation work in their cars.

3. Write for yourself. Don't worry about how your words tumble out, look, or sound. Capture your true thoughts and feelings, questions, and insights. Be sure to highlight any breakthroughs and small steps of progress. You are on your way to living more fully.

Good Grief Vs. Complicated Grief

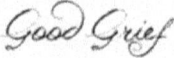

- The common, intensely painful, mental and physical response to loss.
- Intense and dominant thoughts, feelings, and behaviors occur erratically and vary over time
- Blend of yearning and deep sadness
- Shorter attention span than usual
- Accompanying thoughts and memories of the death, and the deceased person
- A tendency to be more interested in your inner world than activities of ordinary life
- Most people move along this painful and challenging road of grief to eventually accept their loss and see a future that has joy and satisfaction. When this transformation does not occur within the first couple of years, reach out for help to prevent Complicated Grief or Prolonged Grief Disorder.

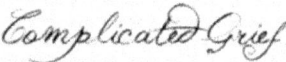

Prolonged Grief Disorder (PGD) exists when 5 or more symptoms are present after six months have elapsed since the loss. The distress causes impairment in functioning socially, on the job, or other areas of responsibility such as home life:

- Confusion about one's role in life or a diminished sense of self
- Difficulty accepting the loss
- Avoidance of reminders of the reality of the loss
- Lowered trust in others since the loss
- Bitterness or anger related to the loss
- Difficulty moving on with life (ie. making new friends, pursuing interests)
- Feeling that life is unfulfilling, empty, or meaningless since the loss
- Feeling stunned, dazed or shocked by the loss
- The distress has been assessed is not a function of major depression, generalized anxiety, or Post-Traumatic Stress Disorder. [8]

3

Your Story Matters

There is no greater agony than bearing an untold story inside you.
Maya Angelou

My husband, John, dashed into the delivery room in his camouflage garb, green paint all over his face, just as Nathan's head was crowning. By now, the drugs they'd given me were working marvelously well, and I was smiling through every contraction. We laughed over John making a typical five-hour return trip from hunting in half the time. Not one of the twelve traffic lights turned red on his way to the hospital. Perhaps angels were flying escort.

Minutes later, our baby boy entered the world. But something was wrong. Terribly wrong.

Our baby was blue, not breathing well, and his little cry sounded muted. Instead of laying him in my waiting arms, the technicians scurried around trying to suction his mouth to help him breathe. John held my hands, and we asked God to help Nathan and to guide the doctors' efforts.

I kept asking the nurses if Nathan was all right, and all I could get out of them was, "He's in good hands, and they're helping clear his passageways." When I asked if I could nurse Nathan, they said they didn't know. An hour later, frustrated with the vague answers and being separated from my son, I asked the delivery nurse to wheel me into the care unit where they were working with Nathan.

The pediatrician on call came over to talk with us. I didn't know this woman, and I didn't want to believe a word she was saying.

"Mrs. Vredevelt, your son is not oxygenating well, so we're trying to help him with oxygen and IVs."

"Is this life-threatening?" I asked.

"It could be," she replied. "It's also my observation that he has Down syndrome. I've called a cardiologist to examine him because his heart isn't functioning properly."

In the shock of it all, I blurted out, "What does this mean?"

"It means he will be mentally retarded, Mrs. Vredevelt, and there is a higher incidence of leukemia among those with Down syndrome. There's a catheter in his heart, and the technicians are still working to stabilize him."

I spent that night alone in my room, listening to happy families around me celebrating their babies. My own personal doctor was in Russia. My pediatrician was on vacation. My parents were in California. John and the kids were home in bed, and a tiny little boy named Nathan Vredevelt was in some sterile room under impersonal fluorescent lights, fighting for his life.

And me? I began to wonder just how much God really loved me.

As hot tears rolled down my cheeks, I remember whispering into the night, "God, what is this? A bad joke? Well, I'm not laughing!"

Words from another time and place passed through my mind, "A bruised reed I will not break and a dimly burning wick I will not extinguish."[32] At the time I couldn't grasp the meaning and didn't have the bandwidth to give it much attention.

The next morning the cardiologist ran a battery of tests on Nathan. Based on the results, he said the center section of Nathan's heart was not formed and he would likely need open-heart surgery when he was closer to four months old. During surgery, he would construct the center portions of Nathan's heart so that he could oxygenate better and follow a more normal growth pattern.

As the cardiologist left the room, anxious thoughts ran wild: What if his heart fails and he doesn't make it four months? What if the surgery doesn't work? What if he gets sick and his body isn't strong enough to fight infection?

How do we raise a child with Down syndrome? What if Jessie and Ben can't adjust to having a handicapped brother? What if…? What if…?

Our family and faith community heard about this chain of events and collectively prayed for Nathan that evening. Within hours, his vital signs took a turn for the better. His oxygenation improved, and by morning, they were able to remove the IV that went directly into his heart. Many prayers continued, specifically for the healing of Nathan's heart.

My mom flew into town to help us. A few days later, we took Nathan to the top-level trauma hospital in Portland, Oregon for more tests. The cardiologist wanted to examine all the cross sections of Nathan's heart using ultrasound to determine how much of the heart muscle needed to be constructed.

We watched the screens intently as the doctor focused on various chambers of the heart. When he got a clear picture of the center section, he started to shake his head and chuckle aloud. I was not amused! Then, in his clipped, British accent, he proclaimed, "By golly, the center of his heart is absolutely normal!"

I cried, my mom wiped tears from her eyes, and the doctor just kept shaking his head in amazement, muttering, "Very good, oh, very good!"

He pointed to a small hole between the upper and lower chambers of the heart and showed us on the screen where blood was spilling through. After taking some measurements, he consulted with us in his office.

"Mrs. Vredevelt," he said, "Nathan has two small holes in his heart. I want to watch these holes carefully for the next six months to see if they will close on their own. If they do, surgery won't be necessary. If they don't close, then we can patch them when he's a little older."

Mom and I continued wiping our eyes while the doctor beamed, telling us how much he enjoyed giving good news.

I left the hospital that day with a renewed awareness: God was still in the business of healing. That truth applied to baby boys with holes in their hearts, and broken-hearted moms and dads with holes in their faith.

Either way, His is the touch that heals.

* * *

Our heart wounds come in all shapes and sizes. Some are forced upon us without a choice. Severed relationships, unwanted endings, shattered plans, broken boundaries, betrayals, debilitating illness—they all come packaged in grief.

Tommy is a tender, innocent seven-year-old little boy. He sees a therapist because his daddy suddenly exploded and walked out on him and his mom a year ago. Tommy hasn't seen or heard from his daddy since.

"Will you draw a picture of your heart for me, Tommy?" the counselor asked.

A bowl of colorful marker pens and white paper sat on the table in front of him. Tommy chose one pen, and colored the entire page completely black, except for one little white square in the middle.

His counselor asked about the tiny white square, and Tommy said, "Oh! That's the way out!"

Similar to Tommy, I believe something inside you senses that there's a way out of your darkness.

I perceived it, too, and I did what many dedicated clinicians would do. I delved into robust scientific research for a more comprehensive understanding of loss, trauma, and grief recovery. I sought God for wisdom, eager to hear Him speak and teach me how to co-create healing practices for mending my broken heart.

Strategic questions begged answers:

- What is my part in the healing process? What is God's part?
- Why are some people able to mend and flourish, when others get stuck or derail the healing process?
- Given similar conditions, what allows one person to rise up strong, while another zombies along for years like the walking dead?

- What practices might promote healing and long-lasting results? What simple routines might revitalize the body, mind, and spirit?

I didn't know, but I was determined to dig deep and see what I could find.

The latest scientific research now supports what many clinicians have suspected for years. *Unresolved loss and trauma can be passed down through generations.*

Leading experts, including neuroscientist Rachel Yehuda[33] and psychiatrist Bessel van der Kolk[34], tell us that even if a disturbing story has been silenced or forgotten, its memory and feelings live on in the body.

Grief imprints our being, leaving effects that often persist for years and decades. Long after the events are over, the body can continue to respond as if danger is ever-present. These emotional legacies are often hidden, and they play a far greater role in our emotional, physical, and spiritual health than what was previously understood.

My professional mission is to help individuals heal their heart wounds using a balanced holistic approach that encompasses the body, soul, and spirit. I have learned that there are personal practices, backed by timeless wisdom and decades of substantial research, that do, in fact, promote emotional healing and greater well-being.

A strategic key to healing after loss is not just knowing what happened to you, but transforming how you remember (how you see, think, and feel about) the losses you've suffered. The ways you tell your story matters, even if you're only telling yourself. More on that later.

I've often wondered: Why don't insights from clinical research seem to move beyond academic arenas to benefit the general public at large? And why are conversations not happening, or at least not easily found, around how clinical and spiritual practices can naturally weave together to promote emotional healing?

Is it really possible to face life's deepest questions—especially around suffering, loss, and even death—without considering the spiritual part of who we are?

I wonder. Can we really make it through these tender, complicated moments without asking God who He wants to be for us, or how He might want to show up in our pain?

And what if… what if loss isn't the end of the story, but something God actually redeems?

Maybe you've wrestled with similar notions. Have you ever caught yourself wanting (or begging, pleading, and demanding) God to change your circumstances? I understand. I have, too.

Often, it seems, God has something far more incredible and comprehensive in mind for us than we do.

Is it possible that in our suffering, God wants to empower change *in* us for a greater good, which custom fits who we were created to be from the beginning, and mirrors our greatest amplitude of being human?

Could it be that God intends to renovate our souls in ways that yield mind-boggling, eternally significant results we can't even fathom?

Emotional healing obviously isn't a clear, straightforward process that happens in a set linear time frame. If it were, everyone who has suffered great loss would eventually thrive. Reality confirms the exact opposite. We all know people who have grown increasingly bitter rather than better over time. Healing your heart takes a very special kind of care and attention.

While there is no going back to the *old you* prior to your loss, a *new you* is currently taking shape. You are different now, and you always have choices. You get to decide where you go from here, the quality of life you want to live, the kind of person you want to be, and the difference you want to make in the future. God is always calling you forward, inviting you higher into your truer self, and more radiant way of being.[35]

The people you love and care about, need the *true* you to show up, not a muted, dim version of you.

They need you to do the productive work of mourning your loss so that you can rise up strong, revitalized, and fully alive. If you have a pulse, you still have significant purposes to fulfill that no one else can.

Fresh exploration and growth opportunities are waiting for you ahead. Take in what is offered, and I believe your days will get a little better than they were before. What allows me to say this with confidence? I've seen it work, in my own life and thousands of others.

Love is stronger than loss.

Record Your Story—Writing to Heal

Are you ready for the next step? It's time to honor your story.

I want to offer you two ways to begin telling your story. Start with the practice you prefer and complete the other one next. Practice #1 uses words to communicate your story. Practice #2 uses creative expression. Ample research verifies that both strategies promote emotional healing and increased well-being.

Read the descriptions of Practice #1 and #2 below. Choose one and begin.

An Invitation to Action: Practice # 1—Tell Your Story

Telling your story is foundational to emotional healing and overcoming your most painful experiences. Immersive, reflective writing helps you pick up the pieces of your broken heart and mend them back together even after the most unimaginable situations.

This practice focuses on recording the memories surrounding the event of your loss. You've likely experienced many losses. Select one that more frequently comes to mind and troubles you in this season.

Please follow these guidelines for writing to heal:

- Write without censorship or evaluation. Grammar and spelling don't matter. What you write does not have to *sound nice* or *make sense*. Grief is messy and that's okay. Advise your inner critic to take a break. Telling your story is safe, productive, and healthy.[36]

- Write freely for 20 minutes and keep your pen moving.

- Write down words and phrases of memories that bubble to the surface related to your loss, both painful and pleasant. There's no need to overthink this. If ideas stop flowing, simply ask God, "What else is important about my story?" and keep writing.

- Record as many details as possible about what happened. Delve into the depth and breadth of the specifics along with your related feelings. Meaning is discovered in the details. There is no right or wrong way to tell your story. Any place is a good place to start. Take your time. Writing your story in a few smaller time segments makes the process easier. Leave blank pages open after your first writing segment, so that you can keep adding to your story as ideas surface. Below are possible questions to help get you started.

Memory Joggers for Writing Your Story:

- What vivid memory stands out from the day of your loss?
- What did you sense, see, hear, taste, touch, smell, and feel at the time?
- When do you remember sensing that something might be wrong?
- What was your first reaction? What followed?
- What did you do?
- Who was available to help?
- What events unfolded within the days and weeks that followed?

REDUCING COMPLICATED GRIEF SYMPTOMS

Studies show that retelling the story of your loss effectively reduces what is reffered to by medical specialists as Complicated Grief. Writing the narrative of your loss, including its associations with other life events, its personal significance and meaning to you, and sharing your feelings with supportive others, has been show to effectively reduce complicated grief symptoms. [37,38]

An Invitation to Action: Practice # 2—Draw a Picture

When heartache overshadows your ability to find words, and you don't know what to say or where to start, drawing is another way to release grief and find peace. There are times when pictures can hold our thoughts and feelings better than words. Creative expression can also provide healthy breaks in the arduous marathon of grief. Relief comes when we fully absorb ourselves in hands-on activity, so much so, that other matters fade into the background.

Brain research shows that activities such as drawing, meditation, reading, music, art, crafts, and other projects stimulate the neurological system and enhance well-being. Creative practices activate the brain's reward system (releasing dopamine), promote relaxation, and quiet the body's fight-or-flight response.

Maddy, a college student, was on a journey of healing with God after experiencing two profound losses. Her mother passed away when Maddy was in first grade, and about ten years later, she lost her father while in high school—both after courageous battles with cancer. The weight of those losses ran deep, and yet Maddy was learning to meet her pain with faith, trusting God to walk her through the healing process.

One of the ways Maddy released her grief was by drawing. Putting her inner world onto paper helped her express emotions that words often couldn't reach—and in those quiet, creative moments, she often sensed God drawing near with comfort and messages of love.

During college, Maddy shared about a day when a wave of anxiety overwhelmed her so completely that she was unable to function. I listened as she gently gave voice to the emotions and memories stirring beneath the surface. Together, we began bringing those hidden parts into the light.

As our time ended, a line in Psalm 23 came to my mind: *"Surely your goodness and mercy will follow me all the days of my life…"*[39] I invited Maddy to contemplate that verse over the coming week, and to capture whatever surfaced in her heart through drawing.

There's more to Maddy's story that I'll share later, but for now, I want to highlight how powerful this simple practice was in her healing. While reflecting on the verse, an unexpected image came to her—one that made her laugh and feel surprisingly light inside. She described it like this:

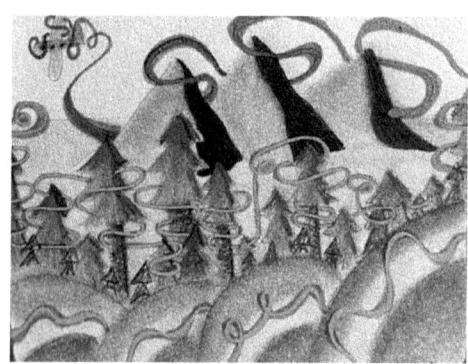

"In my mind, I saw this moving picture that made me laugh—it had a bouncy, fun feeling to it. A purple squiggly ribbon was swishing and swirling through rows of mountains and trees. That swirling ribbon represented the Holy Spirit who felt lighthearted and full of fun. We were in the middle of playing a game and He was chasing after me!

The tall mountains and trees represent the obstacles and struggles I face. But the Holy Spirit was weaving His way through all of it—up and down, over and around—just to stay close to me on the path."

By drawing what she saw, Maddy found a concrete way to lean into grace—especially when she felt most fragile.[40] Revisiting those drawings in the days that followed helped the truth of God's nearness and love take deeper root in her whole being: heart, soul, mind, and body.[41]

Her artwork became more than just creative expression; it was a sacred reminder that the Holy Spirit knew her intimately, understood her burdens, and pursued her with playful, persistent love. Maddy's drawings reflect a deep spiritual truth: that God meets each of us in a deeply personal way—as if we were His one and only love.

* * *

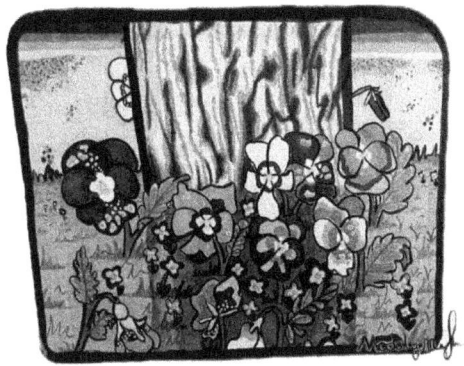

In another quiet moment of prayer, Maddy found herself drawn into a powerful picture. She saw herself standing before the cross, Jesus hanging above her with his arms outstretched in love. One by one, she began handing over her griefs. She gave Him the sorrow of not being able to save her mom and dad, the ache of having to say goodbye too soon. She laid down her fear of more losses, of something else terrible happening, and the deep loneliness that sometimes crept in like a shadow.

As each burden left her hands, she watched them absorb into Jesus' body—disappearing into the mystery of His suffering love. And with each surrender came release. Maddy let go of the pressure to control what couldn't be controlled—the anxious striving to keep her worst fears at bay.

When the last grief had been placed at the foot of the cross, something beautiful happened. A small patch of flowers appeared, blooming at the base. They were delicate and beautiful shades of purple and blue, like Forget-me-nots. These little blossoms seemed to glow with meaning: the enduring nature of love, the sacred memory of those who have gone to heaven, and the invitation to treasure life as it is right now.

In that moment, something clicked for Maddy. With a gentle realization lighting up her face, she said, "God is telling me that He wants me to focus more on the beauty around me, and within me, and even on the beauty that's come out of my pain, instead of letting fear take up all the space in my mind."

It was an amazing shift: from holding on to letting go, from anxiety-ridden sorrow to something priceless that mirrored Triune Love. Allow me to make a disclaimer here. Maddy is a talented young artist, so please, *do not* expect the quality of your drawings to look like hers. The healing path has many important signposts. The marker at this spot reads: NO COMPARISONS ALLOWED.

Think first-grade art. There are no rules, and no one is peeking at your paper. The purpose is to release what is inside.

Your goal is *expression, not perfection.*

On a clean page in your notebook, draw a simple picture of your grief, similar to what a young child might draw. Use markers, colored pencils, crayons, or anything else to capture a visual image of your anguish today. Your picture can be as simple or as detailed as you want.

This is an opportunity for you to listen to your heart and draw what you sense happening on the inside. If you're looking at an empty page and your mind is blank, ask for intuitions of the Holy Spirit to help you with discernment. Divine Light can illumine your heart search.

> *Ever read someone's story and think:*
> *This is exactly what I needed to hear today?*
> *Your story will do that for someone else.*

When your drawing is finished, describe what different parts of the drawing mean in your notebook, along with any before-and-after differences you notice in your heart-soul-mind-body. What subtle shifts or changes are you aware of (physically, emotionally, mentally, spiritually) after expressing your heart in picture form?

Below are sample drawings contributed by people while partnering with God to heal after loss.

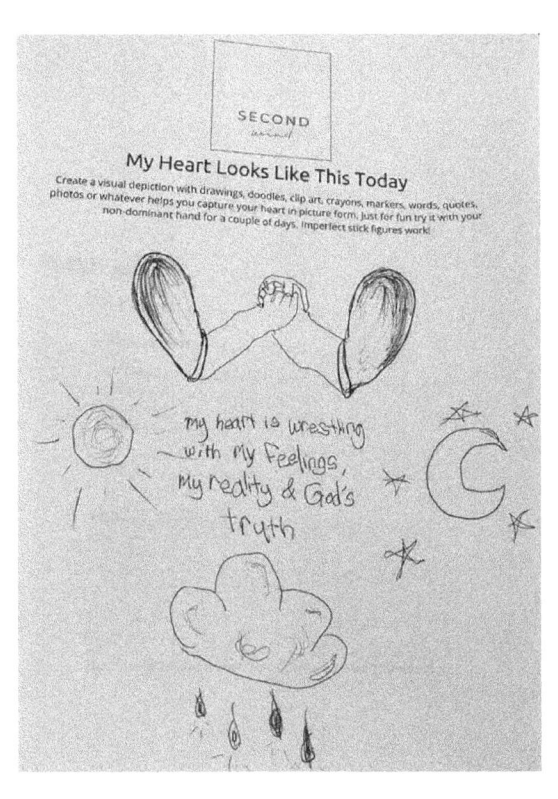

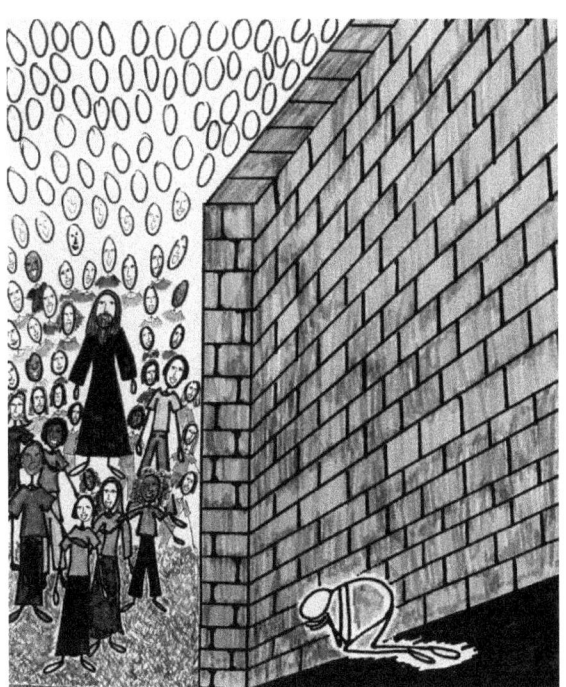

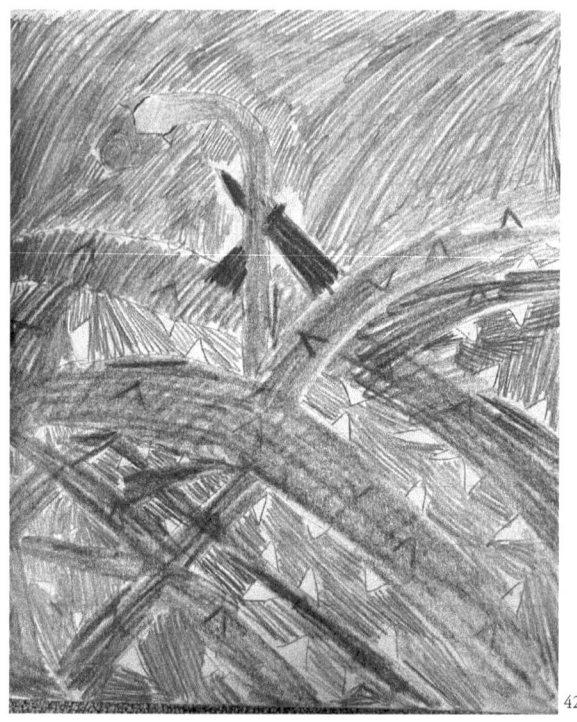

42

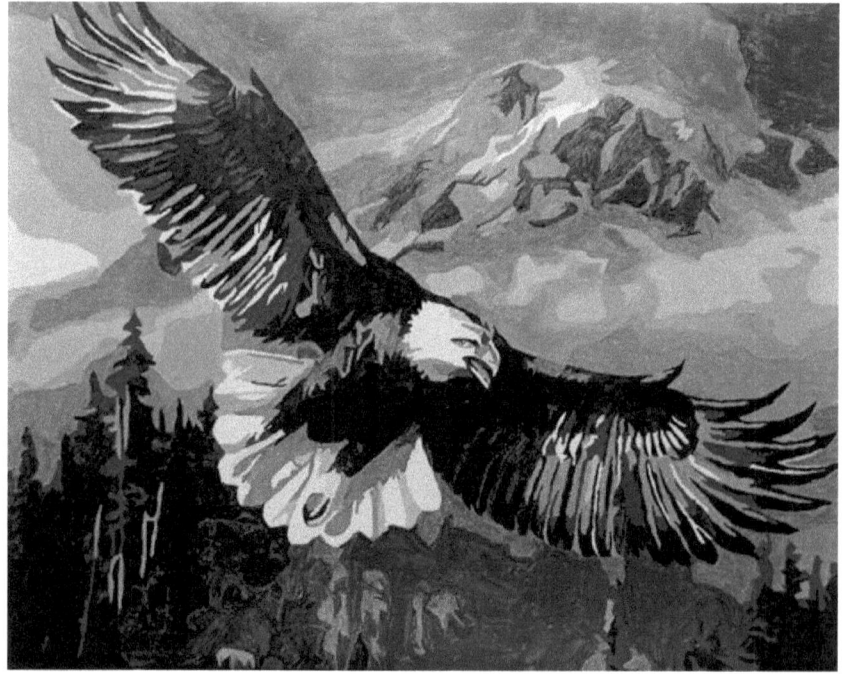

43

An Invitation to Action: Practice #2 (Alternative)—Write a Song of Lament

There are no easy words. No magical expressions to make the heartache of loss vanish. If you prefer not to draw, try writing a poem or song of lament about your loss. This practice promoted healing for our older son, Benjamin. Through creating a song of lament, Ben connected with Nathan, explored meaning, released emotion, and honored the love they shared.

NATHAN'S SONG
© Benjamin J. Vredevelt

Stay close don't ever leave
It's what you would have said.
Now I'm the one who is lonely
Stuck in the middle of life and death.
One-sided conversations are giving me nothing
and testing my faith.
I'm falling over these questions
And searching for answers concerning your fate.

But I will sing about the love, the love you've shown
the love you poured on me
living it out for all to see.
And I will not forget about the times we had
and what you mean to me
I'd give anything for one day but...
If living is Christ and dying is gain
You know I'm not about to get in your way.
I love you so much and I'd like you to stay
But you'll be better off outside of this place.

I know I'm on my way home
I'll just be late.

My refuse to grab my darkest clothes couldn't stop tonight
Now I am feeling the empty spaces you once filled with your life.

So, I will sing about the love you've shown
the love you poured on me
living it out for all to see.
And I will not forget about the times we had
and what you mean to me
I'd give anything for one day…

But if living is Christ and dying is gain
You know I'm not about to get in your way.
I love you so much and I'd like you to stay
But you'll be better off outside of this place.
I've been hurt before but this ain't the same
You've got me burning on the inside today.
I know I'm on my way home

If living is Christ and dying is gain
You know I'm not about to get in your way
I love you so much and I'd like you to stay
But you'll be better off outside of this place
I know I'm on my way home
I'll just be late

Benjamin sang his song with a band at Nathan's Celebration of Life service. Writing the lyrics and charting the instrumentals allowed him to sort through part of his own story and share it with all those grieving Nathan's departure.

Putting words to music is a powerful tool for self-reflection that helps us find words and images to describe our emotions and explore meaning.[44, 45] Poetry and songs have the ability to access our innermost feelings, making it possible to heal emotional wounds no matter how deep they run. The synergy of lyrics and music together slows us down, creating space for us to feel and let go. We can tap into emotions on a deeper level, releasing them, perhaps, in a way we can't experience otherwise.

One of the most heartfelt requests I often receive while speaking at conferences is for access to Benjamin's song. And it's no wonder! Music has a profound ability to help us feel connected, to remind us we're not alone in our experiences. Through its unique artistry, a song can beautifully encapsulate the whirlwind of emotions we all go through, resonating deeply within us. The lyrics and melodies enable us to connect with ourselves, with those who have passed on,[46] and humanity at large. We intuitively sense we're a unique part of something far greater. The healing impact is penetrating and profound.[47]

BENEFITS OF ARTISTIC EXPRESSION

Decades of scientific research-backed evidence reveals the important benefits of creative expression through art:

- Improved well-being, decreased troubling emotions and increased positive emotions
- Improved medical outcomes
- Reduced depression, anxiety, and stress
- Reduced symptoms of compassion fatigue
- Increased healing and sense of purpose
- Improved focus on positive life experiences
- Increased sense of self-worth and social identity

When you finish Practice #2 (the creative expression of a picture, poem, or song of lament), go back and complete Practice # 1 Tell Your Story, as explained above.

An Invitation to Action: Practice # 3—Share Your Story with a Safe Person

Choose someone safe who you believe genuinely cares about you (i.e. a family member, close friend, clergy, or counselor). In the next couple of weeks, take time to connect and read your story to someone you trust. If you're able, share your creative expression, too. It not only supports your own healing, but also helps others by showing what healthy grief work looks like. Healing is most powerful in community.

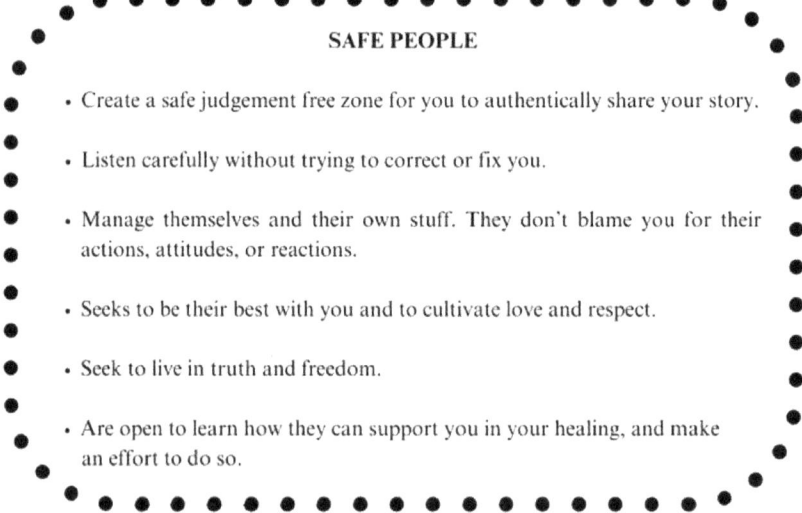

SAFE PEOPLE

- Create a safe judgement free zone for you to authentically share your story.
- Listen carefully without trying to correct or fix you.
- Manage themselves and their own stuff. They don't blame you for their actions, attitudes, or reactions.
- Seeks to be their best with you and to cultivate love and respect.
- Seek to live in truth and freedom.
- Are open to learn how they can support you in your healing, and make an effort to do so.

I've guided countless people through this practice, and time and again, I've seen how sharing their story brings healing. It's rare—almost unheard of—for it not to be a deeply restorative, life-giving experience. Giving voice to our pain and allowing it to be seen is deeply transformative. While a few listeners may not have known how to respond in a supportive way, many others offered kindness, validation, and empathy. In fact, some people said that telling their story led to deeper, more meaningful friendships—opening the door for others to be more honest and vulnerable in return.

Even though reaching out can feel awkward and perhaps even scary, grieving alone is much more risky and it prolongs unnecessary suffering. When you're used to mostly giving, learning to receive requires humility. I'm not saying it's easy or comfortable, but your healing is worth it. It's vital to push the edge of your comfort zone and share your story. Your story matters.

After talking with a safe friend, write a paragraph or two in your notebook about what you experienced while telling your story. Consider these suggestions while summarizing your experience:

- Who did you talk to? Describe their response.
- What benefits came from sharing your story? What was learned?
- What thoughts and feelings do you have about writing and sharing your story?

You don't have to be a professional writer or artist to use writing and drawing as a tool to better understand your experience and find meaning. You simply need to pick up your pen, put it to paper, and then watch your mending unfold.

> *If you don't tell us who you are, someone else might, and get it wrong.*
> *If you don't tell us what you stand for, someone else might, and miss the point.*
> *If you don't put into words what happened, someone else might tell it very differently.*
> *There is power in telling your story yourself.*[48]
>
> Camille DePutter

4

WHERE HEALING HAPPENS BEST

We are what we believe we are.
C.S. Lewis

Most of us land in bewildering desolate places repeatedly during our lifespan. Do you find yourself there now? Feeling alone, abandoned, or forgotten? Do you see yourself spinning in negative loops wondering, "Why am I here? What if I had done this, or hadn't done that? Where did I go wrong? What's the point? Is this all there is? How on earth can I keep going?"

I understand. I really do. I've struggled with similar questions. My training occurred mostly in dismal death valleys, sun-scorched deserts, and long stretches of ambiguous in-betweens. They are not locales I would have chosen for myself. Had I known the script in advance, I might have given up and missed priceless treasures that I wouldn't trade for anything now.

Wrestling is common after a loss. Our greatest battles are often fought within.

This doesn't mean something is wrong with you, or that something in you needs to be fixed. It doesn't mean you have a problem that others don't experience. It simply means your inner world is in confusing disarray because the former shape of your life doesn't match the present.

Loss leaves you dazed and disoriented. Little seems recognizable. You are now in the demanding process of reorienting and realigning your inner world with your altered outer world. This *is* the path of healing.

We typically enter transition zones, nervously clinging to the former shape of things. It's difficult to acknowledge that there's no going back. Our whole way of being is being pressed into a new life pattern. Don't be surprised when you find yourself resisting. It's what we tend to do. Human beings are creatures of habit and most prefer the familiar. I have yet to meet a person who is elated by the ambiguities of being *in between*.

Rest assured, there is much more happening within you than you can possibly grasp right now.

Beyond the visible eye and conscious awareness, the shattered pieces of your heart are reconfiguring into something new and remarkable. Your Creator gifted you with innate abilities to restore, much like you have aptitudes to move, think, and feel.

You may be concerned that this cold, dark season will drag on indefinitely, and that little will ever change. But that's not the way things typically work in our world. Underlying rhythms and natural laws are continuously in motion.

Spring always follows winter.

We witness these mysteries year after year. Suddenly, seemingly out of the blue, new life springs from death. Ancient forests with hollow dead stumps sprout lush ferns and bright flowers. Cheery purple and yellow crocus pierce through soft white blankets of snow. Robins return from the south to nest in decaying old snags. Seasons come and go with built-in exchanges.

As in nature, a transformation of the heart involves intricate creative artistry. Healing is complex, delicate, and s-l-o-w. It requires special conditions, and a masterful guide and guardian to help you mend stitch by stitch. Have you ever considered exploring these mysteries in collaboration with God and safe friends?

Decades of research make it clear: Human beings do not heal well alone.[49]

God was the first to tell us, *It isn't good to be alone*,[50] for the sake of our well-being. We are created to thrive in relationships. Isolation is destructive.

It's a known fact that social isolation significantly increases your risk of premature death from all causes[51], rivaling smoking, obesity, and physical inactivity. It fuels depression, anxiety, and suicide and sets you up for a 50% increased risk of dementia, a 29% increased risk of heart disease, and a 32% increased risk of stroke.[52]

Healing happens best in the context of relationships.

The problem is, that when our hearts are hurting, we tend to pull away and withdraw. After dragging ourselves through basic responsibilities and routines, there's little energy to socialize. We don't feel like interacting or putting on a pleasant face. It feels fake. We don't want to be poor company. Sometimes we're so exhausted we don't care much about anything other than escaping into sleep.

Part of being human is spiritual. We are spiritual beings, created for an intimate and transforming friendship with the creative community that is the Trinity: Father, Son, and Holy Spirit. From my vantage point, optimal restoration and well-being happen best in the context of relationships with God and safe companions.

Will you give yourself permission to try healing practices that include all of you —your body, soul, and spirit? A process that yields enduring results and is far more effective than a shotgun approach to recovery or dismissing your inner truth with toxic positivity. As Tish Warren writes, "When we're drowning, we need a lifeline, and our lifeline in grief cannot be mere optimism that maybe our circumstances will improve because we know that may not be true. We need practices that don't simply palliate our fears or pain, but that teach us to walk with God in the crucible of our own fragility."[53]

What I've come to understand during four decades in the counseling office and my own life journey, is that God is incredibly close to the broken-hearted.[54] Grief opens a door into what the Celtic Christians called a thin place, where the boundary between heaven and earth seems more permeable. We encounter God in fresh ways that startle us out of inattention and transform our ways of being.

Dark nights of the soul provide opportunities to experience God in ways unique to each of us, according to our specific needs, confines, and broader purpose. I've watched this reality play out in countless individuals for over forty years: God can bring about transformation in a brief encounter that might otherwise take weeks or months of personal therapy.

Never underestimate God's ability to communicate with you and provide what you need. He knows how to awaken your mind to what is true, intertwine His thoughts with yours, and help you realign your thinking with His wisdom. In the blink of an eye, he can illuminate obstacles that are holding you back, and free you to get on with life.

When our daughter was 16, between her junior and senior years of high school, she drove the freeway home from the other side of town, after a prep course for college entrance exams. The mid-day traffic was heavy.

She rounded a curve, slowing her speed in sync with the cars in front of her. But the eighteen-wheel truck driver behind her was not paying attention. He slammed into her, crunching the bed of our small Toyota truck like an accordion, to half its original size.

First responders came and examined her. Other than surface burns from the airbag, and a sore neck and back, there were no visible injuries. They advised her to see a doctor for a more thorough exam. Jessie saw a doctor the next day who voiced no major concerns, said her soreness would improve and released her to resume her normal routine.

It didn't take long for us to realize that Jessie wasn't herself.

The following months were miserable. She couldn't read for more than ten minutes without feeling nauseous. Academic work took a nose dive. Rather than consistently attending class, she spent hours sleeping in her car in the school parking lot out of sheer exhaustion. Turbulent mood swings felt like being trapped on a frightening rollercoaster ride she couldn't get off of fast enough.

It was painful to watch and just as baffling. One afternoon, I went for a prayer walk to push the tension out of my body and clear my head. Climbing my way up a steep hill in our neighborhood, tears fell as I poured out my heart: *God, I'm so confused. I don't know what to do. I don't know if I'm doing too much, or too little. I need to know how to help.*

At that moment, an image of a red toolbox, piled high with dozens of tools, appeared in my mind. (The picture carried an element of surprise because tools and toolboxes are not something I typically think about. They fall more in my husband's department.)

A flow of thoughts followed the picture: *Pam, you're just one tool in My toolbox to shape Jessie's life.* The words jolted me like a triple espresso waking my soul from a dull stupor.

I want you to notice the details in this conversation. While venting my confusion, I asked God a specific question about what I could do to help Jessie. God did not answer my question like I had hoped. He didn't tell me what to do.

Instead, God addressed a far deeper need of mine, a blind spot I didn't even know I had. He revealed the crushing sense of over-responsibility I carried about my daughter.

In a lightning-quick flash, the Spirit of God flipped on the high beams to help me see that much of my anguish was fueled by a false assumption that was not true: *Everything is up to me.* God, who understands me better than I understand myself, went straight to the root cause of my overwhelm and freed me from its paralyzing grip.

When our perspective changes, our thinking changes—and with it, the way we live. My transformation wasn't something I orchestrated or controlled. It was God's work in me. This experience is just one example of how we can partner with God to heal our hearts.

Can you imagine the deep relief that washed over me as I began to see our situation from a higher view? In the quiet of a simple twenty-minute walk with God, something sacred happened—a divine exchange.

Moments like these aren't rare when we truly seek God. They can become a meaningful rhythm in your life as well, a practice that gently reshapes how you see, think, and carry what's on your heart.

Experiences like this aren't reserved for a select few. God doesn't play favorites.[55] In fact, it's often our weakness that draws His grace and power the most.[56] No matter where you are or what you're facing, you too can be set free from inner conflicts and unseen entanglements that weigh you down.

After high-school graduation, Jessie was determined to join Youth with a Mission's (YWAM) outreach team in Africa on the Mercy Medical Ship. We were concerned about the health risks. A cardiologist had been closely following her unpredictable bouts of rapid heart rate (150-180 bpm), another lingering effect of the freeway accident. A month before she was to leave, the cardiologist gave her the green light to travel with the group.

Her first week on the Mercy Ship involved intensive training and group prayer. One afternoon the college students and leaders laid hands on Jessie and prayed. She said, "Mom, it felt like God put a finger in my brain and swirled things around, like you stir cake batter with a spoon."

Remember how Jessie was unable to read for more than ten minutes without feeling dizzy and woozy? After the group prayed for her, she read twenty-eight books over the next three months without a hint of nausea. Healing happens best in the context of community.

This part of Jessie's story reminds me of a challenge Dallas Willard offered (and that I took quite seriously) many years ago while studying spiritual formation:

Seek God. Expect experiences.[57]

As I understand it, God's answer to our weariness and turmoil is always, *Come to me*:

> Are you tired? Worn out? Burned out on religion? Come to me. Get away with me and you'll recover your life. I'll show you how to take a real rest. Walk with me and work with me—watch how I do it. Learn the unforced rhythms of grace. I won't lay anything heavy or ill-fitting on you. Keep company with me and you'll learn to live freely and lightly.[58]

It's a compassionate eternal invitation for anyone, anytime, anywhere.

Let's Explore

Can we take a moment to pause together?

I invite you to check in with your body. Do you notice any tension or discomfort—maybe in your shoulders, neck, jaw, chest, or stomach? Are there subtle signs of stress or tightness?

Now, gently turn your attention to your thoughts. Do you sense any resistance or hesitation rising up? Maybe thoughts like, *"I'm not so sure about all this talk about God…"* or *"I started questioning God's kindness and care for me when…"*

Whatever you're noticing—physically or emotionally—it's okay. You're not alone in it. Just take a breath and give yourself permission to be honest about what's coming up.

If you notice any tension, take a few slow, deep breaths. Let your body begin to relax and settle.

There's real value in paying attention to the stress you carry—it offers meaningful insight into what's going on inside you. Becoming aware and emotionally honest about your inner experience is not only healthy—it's a sign of strength. It's what it means to be *real*, rather than pretending, denying, or putting on a brave face.

How you respond to loss can deeply shape what you believe about yourself—and who you become.

When you acknowledge any resistance you're feeling, it can open the door to greater self-awareness. You may begin to understand why you tend to withdraw from God or others, and what beliefs or emotions are driving that response.

This kind of reflection can bring meaning to your experience and uncover hidden assumptions or conclusions you've made about your loss.

If you want to explore what might be fueling your struggle, try asking yourself these three questions:

- What am I believing about myself?
- What am I believing about God?
- What is actually true about this situation?[59]

Now, pause a second. Please read the next line slowly and mull it over.

We don't see things as *they* are. We see things as *we* are.[60]

May I comment on the obvious?

Shut-downs and shut-outs don't solve much of anything.

You have the freedom to believe that life is all up to you and that you're alone on your own. But what if there's another more life-giving choice?

What if the truth is, that you are never alone?[61]

God isn't daunted, disgusted, or disappointed in you for your resistance, doubts, or spiritual conflicts. The same goes for your feelings of shame, guilt, anger, fear, and *anything* attached to those emotions. Yes, anything.

You can keep God at a distance for as long as you choose—but that will never change His unwavering affection for you, or the reality that He draws close to care for you, and compassionately meet your needs.[62]

Nothing in your past, present, or future has the power to diminish God's longing for friendship with you. Let that settle into your heart: God wants you—right here, right now, exactly as you are.[63]

It's simply not in God's nature to stop loving you. He never takes back what He gives, and He never acts in contradiction with Himself. Everything He does flows in perfect harmony with who He is.

So remember this: God doesn't love you because you've changed. He loves you so that you *can* change.

That brings up a meaningful question: *Is it possible for us to grow and become more aware of what's happening within us—and to recognize how God's love is actively working there?*

Yes, friend. Absolutely. And I'd be honored to walk with you and show you what that can look like in your life. But first, please take a moment and respond to the following invitation.

An Invitation to Action

1. Reflect on Your Struggle: Identify the biggest challenge you're facing right now related to your loss. Then, ask yourself these questions about that struggle:

    - What am I believing about myself?
    - What am I believing about God?
    - What is actually true?

2. Anchor Yourself in Truth: Write down the truth you've identified on a sticky note and place it somewhere you'll see it often. Repeat this truth to yourself—think it, sing it, speak it out loud. Review it daily until it becomes a natural, automatic thought. Here's an example of one of my sticky notes:

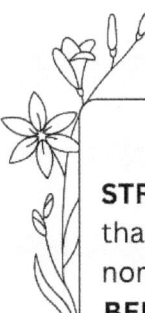

NOTES

STRUGGLE: I'm hollowed out, worried that exhaustion and sorrow are my new normal. Will I ever feel happy again?

BELIEF ABOUT SELF - I feel like I did 3 months ago. Seems like not much is getting better.

BELIEF ABOUT GOD - Will God keep His promise and answer my prayers? I don't know.

TRUTH:

- Negative speculation doesn't help.
- God and I are dealing with my grief together. I'm doing my part. I can trust God to lead me into truth and freedom.
- God hears and cherishes each prayer. Rev. 8:3,4.
- God is renewing my heart-soul-mind-body each day. "You sustain and restore me to full health." Psalm 41:3

5

RESET

*If I had to limit my advice on healthier living to just one tip,
it would be to simply learn how to breathe correctly.*

Dr. Andrew Weil

Breathing is the first thing we do when we are born and the last thing we do before we die, yet most of us pay little attention to it throughout our lives.

We breathe automatically, which is probably why we don't give it much thought. But do you know that slow purposeful breathing is a powerful way to regulate emotions and calm your mind and body?

Your breath is the most effective tool to quickly improve focus, clarity, and intuitive awareness. And it's free.

The word breath in the Bible is fascinating and profoundly symbolic. It implies far more than the physical exchange of air in and out of your lungs. *Breath* in the New Testament Greek language and Old Testament Hebrew dialect means Spirit.

At the beginning of time, the *Spirit* of God hovered over the dark chaos.[64] The Spirit, *ruach* in Hebrew, means *breath,* the creative presence and power of God that brings order to chaos. Out of chaos, Spirit breathed everything into existence bringing forth life, order, and beauty. God formed man, breathed into his nostrils the breath of life, and man became a living creature.[65]

The breath of the Almighty is the life-giving force that not only begins our existence but also gently sustains our body, soul, and spirit. As Job says, *"The Spirit of God has made me; the breath of the Almighty gives me life."*[66] But here's the honest truth: when loss crashes into our lives and shatters our hearts, it can feel like the very breath has been knocked out of us. Grief is not just emotional—it's physical. It can leave us gasping, struggling to find air under the heaviness of pain. Grief can literally take our breath away.

Allow me to review something I mentioned earlier to bring more clarity. E-motion is *energy in motion.* Your body senses this energy in different ways.

The *emotion center* of the brain (known as the limbic system) is located in the back of the brain. It is *much faster to perceive and respond* to incoming messages than the *thinking center* (known as the pre-frontal cortex located in the front of the brain.) The *emotion center* automatically responds at lightning speed to signs of threat or danger without conscious thought or input from you and me.[67]

We don't get to choose our emotional triggers.

When your five senses pick up a threatening signal, *the emotion center of the brain (*in the back) activates a fight-flight-freeze response[68] which, in turn, de-activates the *rational thinking part of the brain* (in the front).

The more stress you carry and the longer you carry it, the more disrupted your nervous system becomes, and the more likely you are to perceive a minor threat as a major danger. An overworked nervous system acts like a faulty fire alarm that sets off ear-piercing sirens screaming to evacuate after lighting a small candle.

Triggered into fight-flight-freeze, your brain releases stress hormones designed to energize you for action. Cortisol and adrenaline pulse through your bloodstream creating physical sensations that tie your gut in knots, cause tension in your shoulders, heaviness in your chest, and a compulsive drive to fight, flee, or freeze in your tracks. Your skin feels cold and clammy, sweaty, or flushed. Your breathing shallows, your mind races, and your thoughts scramble.

This *automatic response* from your *emotion center* is your survival hardware sending a message that says:

1. Something important needs your attention;
2. Engage the thinking center of your brain and be aware of what you sense.

Heightened awareness comes with a regulated mind and body. Clarity, keen focus, and intuitive perception happen best when we are in a settled state of peace.[69]

A question worth considering is: What can we do in real time that is proven to quickly regulate the heart-soul-mind-body out of high alert into calm?

A good place to start is where you did when you first entered this world as a newborn. You breathe, doing what civilizations have done since the beginning of time.

One key to healing your heart lies in understanding and harnessing the power of your breath. Breathing on purpose (B.O.P) activates your body's

God-given built-in relaxation response.[70] Your Creator designed you with an amazing ability to naturally restore balance and quiet your nervous system.

Slow-paced, breathing on purpose is practical and portable. It reduces physical and emotional stress while improving mood,[71] attention[72], and mental acuity.[73]

Drawing from effective practices found in sacred ancient tradition and decades of scientific research, I'd like to suggest three best practices to effectively return to peace and improve awareness when life knocks the wind out of you.[74]

Simple Guidelines to Practice Breathing on Purpose:

#1 Schedule Regular Breaks to Breathe On Purpose (B.O.P.).

> Most of us don't pay attention to how we breathe. However, slow rhythmic breathing acts as a soft reset for your nervous system. Brain changes during slow-paced breathing trigger improvements in awareness and cognition.[75]
>
> Military teams, law enforcement, and first responders use *box breathing*[76] and *tactical breathing*[77] in high-stress situations to improve focus and performance. Stanford University recently released research on *Physiological Sighing,* which includes a double inhale through the nose, the second one shorter than the first since your lungs are already full, and a long, extended exhale through the mouth.[78]
>
> We spontaneously use these sighs without realizing it, in claustrophobic environments or in deep sleep when there is a build-up of carbon dioxide in the bloodstream. This breathing pattern helps offload carbon dioxide while increasing oxygen intake, allowing us to relax. A *few minutes a day* of this sighing

improves mood, decreases anxiety, and reduces respiratory rate better than box breathing or mindful meditation, and the benefits increase over time.[79]

Many slow-paced breathing techniques are available and user-friendly in daily routine. Most encourage longer extended exhales after deep inhales.[80] Free Apps are available to guide the learning process. (iPhone-Deep Breathe; Android-Paced Breathing)

#2 **Breathe through your nose**.

Nasal breathing impacts the central nervous system differently than mouth breathing. Rhythmic nasal breathing paces electrical activity in the brain related to emotion and thought, enhancing perception and memory.[81] It also guarantees a normal supply of oxygen to the brain for optimal performance. On the other hand, mouth breathing interrupts adequate oxygen supply to the brain and can decrease brain function.[82]

The air resistance through nasal breathing increases the vacuum in the lungs and helps us draw in 20 percent more oxygen than through the mouth.[83] Nasal breathing also helps us conserve energy and increases endurance. In contrast, mouth breathing can prematurely shift us into higher energy output, leading more quickly to fatigue.[84] Grieving is exhausting hard work. This is an easy practice to conserve energy for your recovery.

#3 **Try the Ancient Practice of Breath Prayer**

Orthodox tradition says breath prayers originated as long ago as 200 A.D. among the contemplative Desert Fathers and Mothers.[85] While living in barren desolate regions they sought to awaken their attention to God and pray without ceasing.[86] The breath prayer was developed to support the continual awareness of God's presence.

Breath prayer is Scripture-centered prayer used in rhythm with controlled breathing. Your mind focuses on God while you regulate with slow purposeful breathing. Rather than heartache becoming a barrier to your faith, it becomes a portal through which you invite God to join you.

One of the oldest and most common forms of breath prayer is known as The Jesus Prayer. It's fitting, as the signature of Jesus's life was to pursue the downcast and display goodness.

The classical form of the Jesus Prayer says, "Lord Jesus Christ, Son of God," while breathing in through the nose, and exhales saying, "Have mercy on me."[87] The specific words may vary, such as pairing an inhale with, "Lord Jesus" and an exhale with "have mercy." Phrases from the Psalms and other Scriptures are used, as well.[88]

Breath prayer has been used to help people draw near to God when they're spiritually weak. It's a way to confess faith over feelings when the heart is faint, lacking the energy to pray. Rev. John Beck highlights the benefit of this simple prayer:

God sees how we persevere in the struggle, even when our heart is not in it, and God grants the gift of true spiritual prayer, true charity. In a word, God fills us with the gifts of the Holy Spirit… The Jesus prayer promotes confidence in God, trusting that He will see us through times of chaos and tumult, that He will be our Light when we walk through darkness, that He will comfort us in times of illness, spiritual struggle, and distress.[89]

Over time, breath prayer can become as natural as breathing. God's grace gifts ignite hope and build strength. It's one way to prepare for and welcome God's tender care of your grieving heart.

Short Breath Prayer—One to Two Minutes

Option #1—God's Name

God's Name Breath Prayer

Research shows that long, slow exhalations paired with shorter inhalations stimulates the vagus nerve, signaling our nervous systems that we are safe. Breathing on Purpose (B.O.P) helps regulate the heart-soul-mind-body connection and brings balance.

Breath prayer can anchor and support you while breathing on purpose.

Suggestion: Use God's name, Yahweh, which is rooted in the Hebrew letters that compose the English phrase "I AM." The spoken sound of Yahweh mimics breathing.

Inhale through the nose contemplating "Yah" for three seconds.
Exhale through the mouth saying "Weh" for six seconds.
Practice this purposeful breathing for one to two minutes.

*The one thing we do every moment of our lives is . . . speak the name of God.
This makes it our first and last words as we enter and leave the world.
(God's name, Exodus 3:14)
Richard Roher*

Option #2— Two Minutes—Brief Phrases

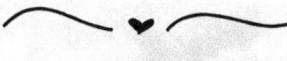

Short Breath Prayer

Choose a phrase to set your focus on God. Match it to your need in the moment. Gently speak the phrase in sync with each slow inhalation (5 seconds) and extended exhalation (7-8 seconds.) Continue for two minutes. Take the liberty to craft your own meaningful contemplations. Here are sample phrases to consider.

INHALE	EXHALE
Holy Spirit	Fill me now
Loving God	You're my peace
Jesus, come	I look to You
You are here	I receive Your love
Spirit of God	Make me new
Perfect Love	I rest in You
I trust You, Lord	I trust You, now

Option #3—5 Minute Breath Prayer

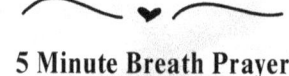

5 Minute Breath Prayer

1 minute: (optional) Set a timer for 1 minute. Bring your notebook and pen to record where and how tension changes in your body before and after this breathing practice. Sit comfortably and imagine yourself in a safe beautiful place, embraced by Love. Slowly, do a body scan, moving your attention from your head down to your toes. Ask yourself:

- Where do I sense tension in my body? (Notice your head, jaw, mouth, neck, shoulders, arms, hands, chest, stomach, legs, feet)
- On a scale of 1–10 (low to high), what level of intensity is the tension now?
- Record the location and intensity of your tension before and after controlled breathing

Example:
Tension – Before: Jaw – 5, Shoulders – 6, Stomach – 3
Tension – After: Jaw – 2, Shoulders – 3, Stomach – 0

***If you are new to breathing practices, this step will give you important information.

5 minutes: Set a timer for 5 minutes. Invite God to fellowship with you. Engage your imagination. See the Author of life sending the breath of His Spirit into your lungs, reviving the wilted places of your soul. Be aware that God is as close as your breath, imparting divine grace to sustain you. Welcome God to open the eyes of your heart. See Him tenderly caring for the shattered pieces of your heart, gently mending and healing. Envision yourself enveloped by perfect Peace and Love while breathing on purpose. Inhale as deeply as you can over 5 seconds and then slowly exhale over 7 to 8 seconds. Continue this for 5 minutes while communing in rhythm with your breathing.
When you become distracted, simply bring your focus back to your breathing and God. Notice what you sense (see, hear, taste, feel, smell) in God's presence.

The goal is to practice regulating your heart-soul-mind-body into a relaxed peaceful state and to record what you sense physically, emotionally, and spiritually.

An Invitation to Action

1. Incorporate breathing on purpose whenever you set aside time to read, reflect and pray.

2. Choose specific times each day to pause and practice intentional breathing. Set an alarm as a reminder. The more you do it, the more natural it becomes—and the benefits grow.

   Some people start and end their day with breathing practice while others use meal times as consistent cues. There's no single right way—just find a rhythm that works for you.

   Once people experience the impact of this simple tool, they often say they won't go without it. It's that powerful. Breathing on purpose creates space for peace, helps you release grief, and opens your heart to receiving God's love.

6

THE POWER OF TRUTH

*I believe that unarmed truth and unconditional
love will have the final word.*

Martin Luther King, Jr.

"I met with two psychics last month. One says my daughter is dead. The other says my daughter is alive, and that I should keep looking for her. People have told me that you're spiritual. I want to know what you think!"

That's how a desperate woman interrupted me fifteen minutes into our first meeting.

I had no information about her background or history. I knew nothing about her values or beliefs. And I had no clue what landmines might be hiding beneath the surface ready to be tripped.

What I did know was horrific. Her daughter, Kari, didn't show up for work one day. Her boss tried multiple times to call Kari and was routed straight to voicemail. It wasn't the first time a college student flaked out on him, but something seemed off. His gnawing gut insisted he reach out to Kari's family.

Mom and Dad hadn't heard from Kari in a couple of days, but that wasn't unusual during the work week. They went to her apartment and discovered her car gone, and that her roommate hadn't seen her for a day and a half. It wasn't like Kari to not come home at night or to miss work.

"She's a good girl. She's responsible, caring, and smart," Mom told me.

A few weeks after Kari went missing, the police discovered a car in a ditch off the side of a back country road. They identified it as Kari's, but no trace of the girl was found near the car.

The police carried out multiple searches to no avail. Professional investigation teams were hired by the family but their efforts led to nothing. The anguish of this distraught grief-stricken Mama tied my stomach in knots.

Her eyes locked hard on mine. This tenacious Mama expected answers. Her suffering was palpable, and I wanted to be very careful with her heart.

My body was on high alert, not having been in a place quite like this before. It's hard to think clearly when you're amped up. Words are much easier to find in the calm.

"You're shouldering the weight of extreme trauma. Let's pause a moment and take a few deep breaths," I replied.

We filled our lungs with air, and I silently prayed for wisdom.

I was reminded that God is very close to the broken-hearted. He created and cherished this woman. The compassion I felt for her was minuscule compared to the immensity of God's kind-hearted love that brought us together.

"Laura, I'm sorry you've received conflicting answers that have intensified your confusion. I do not know whether your daughter is alive or dead. But I can tell you how you can find your answer."

Bewilderment spread across her face. Widened eyes peered at me waiting.

"God is here with us right now. If you want to, you can ask the Spirit of the Living God to tell you the truth."

"I don't know how to do that," she said. "Can you help me?"

"Sure, I can help you," I replied. "We can talk to God, like we talk to a friend, and invite God to show us the truth. Would you like to do that together?"

"Yes," she nodded, "I would!"

I led her through a brief prayer where she repeated short phrases after me. I don't recall our exact words, but it was something simple like, "Spirit of the Living God, I need help. I want the truth about my daughter. Will you please help me?" It was simple.

She opened her eyes, exhaled a huge sigh, and said, "I feel peace."

I encouraged this brave Mama to intentionally watch for ways God might communicate with her: "Specific words or pictures may come to your mind. New ideas may surface. Circumstances may line up in ways they haven't before. God's presence goes with you when you leave here. You aren't alone. Will you keep a record of what you sense God communicating to you?"

She agreed to do so and scheduled another meeting.

I thought often about this courageous Mama in between sessions. I wasn't sure how the Truth would show up, but I knew deep inside that God wouldn't let her down. I trusted God to come through for her somehow, someway.

That confidence stems from my belief that God is always with us, and in knowing we have been designed with an ability to connect with God anytime we choose. The problem is, we often don't pause or take time to be aware of God or to notice the ways He reveals his presence. We forget to tune in, to ask questions, and to listen. So many other loud voices distract and preoccupy our attention. But that can change. We can be more on the lookout for how God is working in our lives.

Brave Mama and I met by teleconference a couple of weeks later. I noticed a different energy in her eyes than before. She leaned in toward her computer and said, "You aren't going to believe it. Something crazy happened!"

I braced myself, wondering what that "crazy" might be.

She said that a policeman called to tell her that a hiker had reported an incident. He was walking along the lake when a slight movement off to the left caught his attention. A damaged old dock was floating against the bottom of a cliff at the water's edge. He left the path, scaled down the bank for a closer look, and happened to notice something hung up under the dock beneath the water. The officer wasn't certain, but he thought the hiker may have found her daughter's body. He would know more after receiving the test results. Shortly thereafter, his hunch was confirmed.

Three years after her daughter disappeared, and two weeks after Mama invited the Spirit of the Living God to tell her the truth, a hiker just happened to notice something in the water. Little did he know the rippling impact his curiosity would have on the storyline of a family that shared similar features to his own. His "chance" sighting that day *just happened* to be the raw material of God's redeeming love. A love that closed an unsolved mystery and ended a mama's heart-wrenching search for her missing daughter.

It is often through great mystery that truth is revealed. What strikes me is how God accompanied this strong Mama straight into her deepest darkest fear, and settled her heart with tangible peace, before she ever left our meeting or had answers. It is often the most painful areas of our lives that we neglect and avoid, where God waits to meet us.

The role of truth is central to spiritual formation, writes John Mark Comer. It undermines untrue stories we believe; it says, "This is true, and this is a lie." It shifts our trust. It rewires our mental maps to reality making it possible for us to live in alignment with reality in such a way that we flourish and thrive according to God's wisdom and good intentions.[90]

Though the truth was deeply painful, it gently freed this brave Mama from the grip of fear—especially the fear of the unknown. It brought a quiet sense of closure and stirred a new courage within her… the kind that comes when you realize you're not walking alone. With God's hand in hers, she found the strength to take one small, brave step forward on the path of healing.

Even the smallest step in the right direction is still a step forward.

When we dare to embrace the truth, even when it hurts, it opens the door to a deeper freedom—the kind that heals from the inside out.[91]

An Invitation to Action

1. Write honestly about one issue you're struggling with today. Use your journal to freely express your thoughts and emotions—no need to filter, judge, or fix anything. Just let it out.

2. Pause and quiet your mind. Ask God: "What is a healthy way for me to see this? What's Your perspective?" Take time to listen with an open heart.

3. Write down any thoughts, feelings, or insights that come to you. Over the next few days, stay alert to anything that connects with this prayer—new understanding, peace, or unexpected clarity. Come back to your journal and add those reflections.

One day, you will tell your story of how you overcame what you went through, and it will be someone else's survival guide.

7

WHAT'S THE BIGGER PICTURE?

Lord, stamp eternity on my eyeballs.
Jonathan Edwards

Shortly after we came home from the hospital with our son, Nathan, our friend, Kay, called. "I'm coming over to clean your house," she said. "What's a good day?"

She showed up on our doorstep a couple of days later with Idella, another friend we'd known for years. What a sight greeted my eyes when I opened the front door. These two looked like they'd just stepped off the set of a Sci-Fi movie with buckets on their heads, gas masks on their faces, combat boots, striped socks, and aprons to cover crazy-looking outfits that you and I would have sorted and pitched thirty years ago.

They came to make me laugh. It worked! But Kay and Idella's visit was far more significant to me than the laughter—or the clean floors and dusted furniture they left behind. I'd known Kay and her family for many years. Kara, their youngest, was born with cerebral palsy and had endured multiple extensive surgeries. For twelve years, Kay had walked a path I was just beginning.

When I saw her standing there in that wild getup on my porch, smiling from ear to ear, I remembered the many times I'd seen her in the past and thought, *She has such heavy burdens. How can she be so happy?*

I plopped myself in our big stuffed chair in the living room to nurse Nathan and said, "Kay, I'm struggling with something. I don't know how to make peace with Nathan's Down syndrome. What helps you?"

Wise lady that she is, Kay didn't offer pat answers or simple platitudes. Instead, she pointed me to a story that had been meaningful to her after Kara's birth. It went like this:

Walking down the street, Jesus saw a man blind from birth. His disciples asked, "Rabbi, who sinned: this man or his parents, causing him to be born blind?" Jesus said, "You're asking the wrong question. You're looking for someone to blame. There is no such cause-effect here. Look instead for what God can do."[92]

God spoke to me on that brisk fall afternoon. He challenged me to shift my focus—to quit trying to "figure it all out." To stop asking "Why?" and instead lift my eyes to God to watch and listen.

Look instead for what God can do.

I pondered those words for a long time while cradling Nathan that day. I wondered about the blind man before he met Jesus. Life as he'd always known it was one long endless night. I'm guessing he never imagined it would be any different, or that his story would become historically significant, or that he'd testify to the governing powers of the day about his radical transformation. Mull that over.

No one knew that one day he'd pull up a seat around a campfire with his family and friends, and tell the story of how God opened his eyes to a brand-new way of seeing.

Who can give you and me the ability to believe we have a future that's brighter than the darkness shrouding our loss?

God.

And who can give you and me the faith to believe our lives and family are in God's hands…no matter what?

God.

Who can give us the faith to believe God is leading us out of the darkness of grief's crevasse when circumstances seem to point another direction?

God.

God challenges you and me to have eyes of faith for ourselves, our relationships, our assignments, and our aspirations. He knows the deepest desires of your heart, what will most satisfy you, and the best ways to help you move from point A to point B.

God's timeless promise still stands: *For I know the plans I have for you… They are plans for good and not for disaster, to give you a future and a hope. In those days when you pray, I will listen. If you look for me wholeheartedly, you will find me.*[93]

God—with full awareness of our weaknesses, wounds, handicaps, and disappointments—challenges us to place our trust in Him…*even when our hearts are breaking…even when our logic screams that He doesn't care or that He has made a terrible mistake.*

In our most fragile moments, we're faced with a sacred choice. We can close off our hearts in bitterness and pain—or we can bravely open the wounded places to God and invite Him in. When we choose to let Him enter our sorrow, He doesn't come with judgment or shame. He comes with tenderness, with compassion, and with healing in His hands.

Gently, over time, He begins to mend what's been broken. He takes even our deepest pain and lovingly weaves it into something far more beautiful than we could ever imagine. There is no wound too deep, no weakness too great, to keep God from fulfilling His purpose in your life. In fact, the very places we see as limitations are often the ones where His grace and power shine the brightest.

That sacred invitation to trust changed the way I saw everything—including our special son, Nathan. Nathan, with his radiant smile and Down syndrome, is not a mistake. He is a masterpiece, a one-of-a-kind work of art, crafted by the hands of a loving Creator for a divine purpose.[94] I believe with all my heart that Nathan walks a path designed especially for him—one full of meaning, beauty, and grace.

And you, my friend, are also *who you are* by divine design. And with that divine design comes very good, significant assignments that only you can fulfill.

Sometimes I wonder what I'll say when Nathan is old enough to ask about his Down syndrome. What words will I have when the world isn't kind—when bullies call him names like "retard" or "misfit," or worse, suggest he's some kind of mistake? What will I say to our beautiful boy?

I imagine pulling him onto my lap, wrapping him up in my arms, and saying something like this:

"Nathan, I want you to know something really important. You are one-of-a-kind, wonderfully made exactly as you are. God dreamed you up and called you into this world with purpose. You're not here by accident. You came at just the right time, to just the right family, because you have a light in you that this world needs.

"Even before I felt you growing inside me, God knew you. You were already in His heart, already deeply loved. You're not an afterthought, Nathan. You're chosen. You belong—to God, and to us.

"You are a joy and delight. When God looks at you, He smiles, like we do. Sometimes people get cranky when things take you a little longer. But Nathan, everyone has strengths and weaknesses. You shine in ways other's don't.

"You're happy—really happy. You give the biggest bear hugs. You light up a room with your laughter, and you love people so easily. That's a gift, Nathan. Not everyone knows how to do that. But you do, and it's something special that you offer the world.

"You're also strong in spirit. You have a beautiful ability to see things other people miss. The way you see angels is amazing. Your name, Nathan, means 'the gift of God.' Your middle name, Charles, comes from my father, your Grandpa Walker. It means *spiritual perception* and your life displays this gift.

"God has already done miracles in your life. When you were born, your heart was broken. There was a hole in it, and we didn't know if you'd make it. But people prayed, and God healed you. You're here for a reason, Nathan, and I believe that reason is full of purpose and love.

"So, when someone says something that hurts, I want you to remember the truth: you belong to God, and to us, and you are deeply loved. We'll talk about the hard things, we'll pray together, and we'll look for what God is doing—even when life is hard and your heart is hurting."

Friend, let this gentle reminder bring comfort: God showed up for a man born blind, and for countless men and women through the ages whose hearts were broken, and who longed for something more. He's shown up for our little boy, Nathan. And God will show up for you, for me, and for anyone who's willing to look for Him.

More often than not… you find what you're looking for.

An Invitation to Action

1. Grief can cloud your perspective and color your days gray. Ask God to open the eyes of your heart to help you see His goodness and love—in the world around you and within your own soul.

2. Practice "Three Good Things." Grief often pulls our minds toward the negative. Before you go to sleep, write down three good things you noticed during the day. Keep it simple—things like the scent of a flower, the warmth of sunlight, laughter, a kind word, or a moment of peace. Anything that gently awakened one of your senses. Whisper a prayer of thanks as you turn out the lights.

3. Name your strengths. Write down three of your greatest strengths. They can be character traits, abilities, or values that define you. Invite two or more people who love you to share what they see as your top three strengths. Jot down their answers, then combine them with your own list. Dedicate a page in your journal titled **MY STRENGTHS**. Add your list and decorate the page. Let it remind you that you are deeply loved, uniquely made in God's image, and created for purposes designed especially for you.

8

THE SECRET OF SURRENDER

If you want change, you have to begin with the man or woman in the mirror.

Eric Metaxas

After Nathan came home from the hospital, I struggled with overwhelming grief driven by postpartum hormones, anxiety about the holes in my baby's heart, and my inability to be the wife and mother I had been before.

Two months after Nathan was born, I stood in the shower, blubbering about it.

"I am so sick of crying, God. I've cried every day for the last two months, and I'm SICK of it. I can't fix me. I can't fix my family. I can't fix Nathan.

God…I need help. Scripture says that You can turn mourning into joy. God, would You please do that for me? Because—no matter how hard I try—I can't do it myself."

I call that ten-minute episode "Surrender in the Shower." It was a turning point for me.

- I surrendered to the fact that I was powerless to change Nathan's condition. I couldn't rewrite the script, nor could I erase the last year of my life.

- I surrendered to the fact that I wasn't capable of meeting my husband's and children's needs the way I wanted to. God knew that, too, and He was going to have to make up the difference.

- I surrendered to the fact that I couldn't control the future. It was in God's hands.

- And I surrendered to the fact that my feelings were my feelings—and in spite of the pain and confusion they created, I knew the only way to freedom was to acknowledge, feel, and ride them out. In that process, I could trust God to partner with me and orchestrate the way to heal my broken heart.

There's nothing like a word of encouragement that drops in your lap, at the precise moment you need it most. I keep a file of God Notes that have arrived right on time. One message enclosed a clipping from the newspaper that challenged me to open my heart in a new way to the direction my life had taken.

It helped me see that much of my anguish was caused by my own resistance.

Being in a tug of war with the events or circumstances in our lives does not change things. Our reality is what it is. Trying to escape or leave the present doesn't help either. But I know something that *does* help.

Acceptance.

Acceptance doesn't make things harder; it makes them easier.

It empowers us to see with a new set of eyes.

I am often asked to describe the experience of raising a child with special needs —to try to help people who have not shared that unique experience to understand it, and to imagine how it would feel.

Emily Perl Kingsley said it beautifully in a little story she penned years ago. She begins by saying that when you're going to have a baby, it's like planning a fabulous vacation - to Italy.

"You buy a bunch of guidebooks and make your wonderful plans. The Colosseum. Michelangelo's David.

"After months of eager anticipation, the day finally arrives. You pack your bags and off you go. Several hours later, the plane lands. The flight attendant comes in and says, 'Welcome to Holland.'

"*Holland?!*' you say. 'What do you mean, Holland? I signed up for Italy! I'm supposed to be in Italy. All my life I've dreamed of going to Italy.'

"But there's been a change in the flight plan. They've landed in the Netherlands and there you must stay. The important thing is that they haven't taken you to a horrible, disgusting, filthy place, full of pestilence, famine, and disease. It's just a different place.

"So, you must go out and buy new guidebooks. And you must learn a whole new language. And you will meet a whole new group of people you would never have met.

"It's just a *different* place. It's slower paced than Italy, less flashy than Italy. But after you've been there for a while and you catch your breath, you look around…and you begin to notice that the Holland has windmills…and Holland has tulips. And Holland even has Rembrandts.

"But everyone you know is busy coming and going from Italy…and they're all bragging about what a wonderful time they had there. And for the rest of your life, you will say, 'Yes, that's where I was supposed to go. That's what I had planned.'

"And the pain of that will never, ever, ever, *ever* go away…because the loss of that dream is a very significant loss.

"But…if you spend your whole life mourning the fact that you didn't get to Italy, you may never be free to enjoy the very special, the very lovely things…about Holland."

I had occasion to think about that "unintended Holland trip" when I found myself sitting at a preschool classroom table with my knees in my throat. Preschool chairs are not made for adult women five feet seven inches tall.

But it didn't matter. This was a special occasion. Our youngest son, Nathan, had invited me to a Mother's Day tea. It had been years since I attended my first celebration as a mom. I remember watching our first-born daughter, Jessie, in her pink polka-dot dress and blond ponytail sing the special music just for Mom. With total confidence, she stood in the front row and belted out the songs at the top of her lungs. Watching her sing I thought, *She's so bubbly and full of life. None of this intimidates her.*

Then there was the time our second born, Ben, played Joseph in the kindergarten Christmas program. He was given the assignment of pulling Mary, who was inside a cardboard donkey which she carried around her waist, several times around the stage. This was supposed to represent their long journey to Bethlehem.

The teacher had told them to park the donkey stage left before walking over to the manger, stage right. When Ben (Joseph) tugged on the rope to park the donkey as per instructions, however, he hit a snag. Mary, with a mind of her own, assertively leaned back in her donkey, refusing to budge.

But Joseph was a man on a mission and he wasn't about to be bullied. So, he hauled off and gave a turbo-charged yank on the rope, which propelled a startled Mary three feet forward. Infuriated, Mary threw down her donkey, slammed her hands on her hips, gave Joseph a *very* dirty look, and stomped offstage.

Ben (Joseph), stunned by Mary's unpredictable mood swing, stomped over to the manger, crossed his arms in defeat, and planted a huge pout on his face. And so goes the story of Mary and Joseph's first fight. So much for an angelic nativity scene.

Many times, I've watched Jessie and Ben on stage, laughing and crying awash in waves of love, soft touch that I am. After the formal presentations, they usually served me coffee and cookies and guided me around the classroom to see what they had made for the occasion. They were proud I had come and proud I was their mom.

This time around, I knew it would be different. This time it would be Holland, not Italy.

I knew Nathan wouldn't be able to articulate the words of the songs and would probably miss some hand motions here and there. I knew that twenty other mothers in the classroom might upset his predictable routine and shake his confidence. I wasn't at all sure how the morning would go…but I made an important decision before I ever walked through that classroom door.

I decided to open my heart to whatever was ahead and to accept it the best I could with gratitude.

Surrendering expectations is powerful.

It brings quiet peace to a heart torn with conflict. It comes when we make a simple choice to take a deep breath and say, "We are exactly where we are supposed to be at this moment in time."

It means we stop wasting precious time and emotional energy wishing things were different, or longing to be someone else, or wanting another set of circumstances.

It's a force for change that can turn bad into good.

It's trusting that all my moments are held in God's loving hands.[95]

The circumstance doesn't matter. It may be singleness. Or widowhood. A heartbreaking marriage. An estranged relationship. Infertility. Disease or disability. Lingering illness. Or *any* life situation in which we find ourselves and over which we have no control.

Finding peace and healing is learned through experience.[96]

When the children presented their songs at teatime, Nathan stood at my side and made his best effort to say a few syllables. His hand motions weren't well-defined, but they were consistent. His pudgy little hand gripped my shirt, and he smiled much of the time. He was enjoying this!

During one of the songs, I glanced at another mom who happened to be watching Nathan. She had sad tears in her eyes. I'm not sure what she was thinking, but a spontaneous insight bubbled to the surface at that moment.

I realized I was in a *different place*, and not one of my choosing. That much was clear. But I also realized that *God* was also in this different place with me. He and I were in this together... for the long haul.

After the presentation, I took Nathan by the hand and guided him around the room to view his artwork on the walls. I pointed to his pictures and said, "Very nice, Nathan!" And then he proceeded to bring me one cookie after another from the silver tray. Between the two of us, we must have eaten a dozen. The limit was two. Oh well.

A deep sense of gratitude welled within as I left the school that day—gratitude to God for helping me move through years of heartache, and for teaching me the secret of surrender.

That doesn't mean I don't feel sad now and then. I do.

That doesn't mean I never play the "What if?" game. I do.

That doesn't mean I never daydream about "Italy." I do.

But less now. Less than before.

I am grateful that God has taught our family to perceive Nathan's differences as unique gifts to be appreciated and understood. I am grateful that the joy over what Nathan can do far surpasses the sadness over what he cannot do.

But most of all, I am grateful that "the handicapped boy in the class" (as some refer to him) belongs to me, and that he's proud I'm his mom.

There's a lot of love in Holland.

An Invitation to Action

1. Are you wasting time and emotional energy wishing things were different, longing to be someone else, or wanting another set of circumstances? Record three or more truth statements to rehearse the next time you start slipping into that bottomless pit.

2. Grief tells us what we can't control, what is missing, and what we cannot do. Write three to five truth statements in your journal about what you can control, what you *do* have, and what you *can do*.

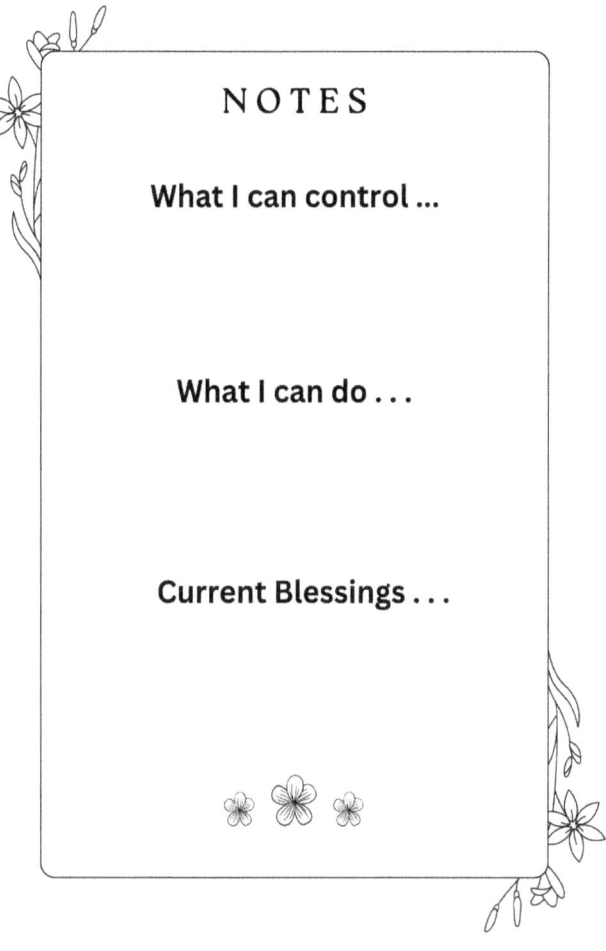

NOTES

What I can control…

What I can do…

Current Blessings…

I'm now in the middle of a fierce battle with cancer. After an MRI, I made the incredibly hard decision to pack up my things and drive 17 hours to another state for treatment. That meant leaving behind my amazing husband and our four young children—for an unknown length of time.

Most of my life I've lived in fight or flight mode, with a deep-seated belief that if I could control my surroundings and outcomes, I'd prevent myself from being deeply hurt again. With so much out of my control—our finances, my lodging, and the emotional toll this was taking on all of us—I cried out in desperation: God, what does it actually look like to completely trust You?

In that moment, a verse from Proverbs came gently but clearly to mind: "She will laugh without fear of the future."[i]

With tears streaming down my face, I told God, "I'm taking my hands off everything. I trust You with it all." And I meant it. I let go of the heavy burden I'd been carrying, hugged and kissed my family goodbye, and, through tears, pulled out of our neighborhood to begin the long journey across the country.

I made a promise to God as I drove that I wouldn't book a single place to stay unless He clearly led me to it. And with that, a deep peace settled over me—the kind that comes when you finally stop trying to direct outcomes and instead, let God be God.

On the second day of my drive, I got a call from a friend. She told me someone we both knew recently moved where I was headed. "They live ten minutes away and have a room with a private bathroom ready for you." Her call brought a flood of tears. I had specifically asked God for a private bathroom—and He didn't miss that detail. He saw me. He heard me. And He provided.

Since then, people I've never met—and others I barely know—have supported our family. As I continue treatment, we're trusting God to meet all our needs, day by day.

Through these challenges, I've learned something I didn't fully understand before: peace and safety don't come from striving to control. They come from letting go—from releasing every detail to the One who already sees the whole picture, and who loves us more than we can comprehend.

God is showing me—over and over again—that I can trust Him.

(1) Prov. 31:25, NLT

LOVE TALK

Elona

9

RECOGNIZE WITH COMPASSION

Self-rejection is the greatest enemy of the spiritual life because it contradicts the sacred voice that calls us the "Beloved." Being the Beloved constitutes the core truth of our existence.

Henry Nouwen

When the shock of a traumatic incident or sudden loss wears off, the implications of what has happened assault your senses with emotional overwhelm.

Some refer to this natural phenomenon as *backdraft*. It's a firefighting expression that describes what happens when a door in a burning house is suddenly opened. Oxygen swooshes in and flames rush out.

A similar process occurs when shock fades away and we open our hearts to compassion—love blows in and the pain rushes out.[97]

Grief is not neat and tidy. It's messy and complex, especially when unpredictable circumstances pull the rug out from under you and land you in a prolonged season of suffering.

The truth is you are a one-of-a-kind treasure, called by name, and deeply loved by your Maker. God created you intrinsically lovable. God *is* love and he always acts in alignment with who He is.

Here's the rub. You've been surrounded all your life by cultural voices that have countered your true identity with lies. Critics within and without murmur that you're not worth much, you aren't good enough, don't have it together, you're different, and don't belong. When adversity throws you into grief, your natural human inclination is to believe and focus on this rubbish.

Do you know that negative thoughts stick in the brain like Velcro and positive thoughts slip away like eggs off Teflon?[98] This hard-wired bias is what allows us to easily detect danger, take action, and survive as a species.

Legitimate grief coupled with this negativity bias, pulls us unwittingly into harmful, dark thought loops. Don't be surprised if you find yourself repeatedly overthinking and ruminating on fear-guilt-or-shame-filled scenarios. Becoming aware of these damaging spin-cycles is the first step to rising above and beyond them. In St. Teresa of Avila's words, "Almost all problems in the spiritual life stem from a lack of self-knowledge."

In 1530, John Calvin wrote, "Our wisdom… consists almost entirely of two parts: the knowledge of God and of ourselves. But as these are connected together by many ties, it is not easy to determine which of the two precedes and gives birth to the other."[99]

Self-awareness is key to emotional healing.[100]

When you criticize, condemn, and reject yourself, you become both the attacker and the attacked. This activates your fight-flight defenses, and dumps stress hormones into your bloodstream, putting you on high alert. Linger in hypervigilance for extended periods and all sorts of health problems show up.

Is it any wonder that our raw anguish attracts divine affection? God draws near to the broken-hearted.[101] Like an attentive mother captivated by her baby's cries, God cannot bear to keep his distance from our weakness and pain.[102] He loves us way too much to stay away.[103] Even when we're not aware of God's imminence, or we conclude He's checked out and doesn't care, Love's presence is no less real.

Do you know the first word God uses when He describes His nature? In the most quoted verse of the Hebrew Bible, God explains who He is: "The Lord, the Lord, the compassionate and gracious God, slow to anger, abounding in love and faithfulness…"[104]

The first quality at the top of the list defining God's character is *compassion*. The Hebrew word for compassion, *rakhum*, comes from the root word, *rakhem*, meaning, womb. Think of God's compassion as womb-like, able to hold, carry, nurture, and protect the sacred life known as *you*. Where empathy says, *I feel you*, compassion says, *I hold you in your pain*.

Compassion is an intense emotional word, often used to describe God's heartfelt response to human suffering. It's an action word that depicts God's inexhaustible energy moving him to rescue those He loves, as a devoted parent saves a child trapped in trouble. It's not a temporary mood, but a fixed attribute of God's eternal being.[105]

In the Gospels, the word compassion, *splanchnizomai,* in Greek, is mentioned more frequently than any other word that identifies the feelings of Jesus. It reflects the gut-churning emotion Jesus felt when he met those who were suffering such as the grieving mother who lost her son,[106] the harassed and helpless,[107] the blind,[108] lost, and the weary.[109] Compassion compelled him to soothe, deliver, and heal.[110]

Learning to care well for your heart, in essence, aligns you with the Source of all compassion.

Healing happens best rooted and grounded in love.[111] Just as you cannot live without water, you cannot mend your heart without compassion. But *with* compassion, you are capable of so much more than you can possibly imagine.[112]

John O'Donohue, an Irish poet and Priest, views self-compassion as the mirror of our lives lived in authentic relationship with God. "There is a place," he says, "that is the eternal place within you. The more we visit there, the more we are touched and fused with the limitless kindness and affection of the divine…If we can inhabit that reflex of divine presence, then compassion will flow naturally from us."[113]

Love is the power source for healing your wounds. In an atmosphere of loving-kindness, you gradually mend and become more inclined to give away what you have freely received.[114]

Science backs what God has said all along. Do you know that the presence of compassion deactivates threats and stimulates the reward center of the brain? It also decreases muscle tension, lowers cortisol, and regulates your heart, while increasing positive mood and overall well-being.[115]

We are designed to thrive in an environment of compassion, not hostility.

Let's bring this down to daily life. Have you ever noticed a difference between what you silently say to yourself when you're hurting, and what you openly say to a friend who is sad or troubled? Perhaps like many with whom I've talked, self-blame, judgment and criticism fill your thoughts far more than compassion. We tend to be harsher toward ourselves than we are with others.

Therapist Warning: Your heart cannot heal in an atmosphere of coarse criticism and condemnation.[116] It's critical to create a judgment-free, truth-telling zone in alignment with God's love.

Rather than avoiding or disconnecting from grief, we choose to compassionately partner with God *through* our sorrowful transitions toward abundant wholeness.

If, by chance, you're worried that self-compassion leads to selfish or narcissistic tendencies, let me ease your mind. Research shows that those who practice self-compassion actually increase their capacity and motivation to help others who suffer. They're also far less prone to depression and anxiety,[117] and more likely to experience post-traumatic growth.[118]

I'm often asked: *What does self-compassion look like in everyday life?*

Imagine yourself caring for a child or elderly loved one who is sick with a fever. What do you do? You approach them gently, speak softly, and explore ways to make them more comfortable. You bring them fresh water, encouraging small regular sips. When they're able to eat, you offer healthy nourishing food.

You find ways to reduce their distress. Expectations around typical responsibilities are laid aside. You encourage rest to conserve their energy for getting well. Your main goal is to bring relief and provide what they need to overcome their illness.

A similar approach is needed to recover emotionally and re-awaken to life after loss. We must come to know ourselves well and learn to love ourselves as God does. Hear the wisdom of Augustine from 400 AD, "How can you draw close to God when you are far from your own self? Grant, Lord, that I may know myself that I may know thee."[119]

On that note, allow me to highlight two non-negotiable basic necessities for your heart to mend.

- *Slow down, so you don't break down.* Conserve energy. Refuse to push hard and fast, rather than white-knuckling it through the day. Quickly respond to your body's legitimate needs: signals of pain, tension, hunger, thirst, and fatigue.

- *Be soft and gentle with yourself.* Kindly accept your heartache as part of being human.[120] Lighten your load. Find ways to release yourself from unnecessary expectations and demands.

Healing Practice: Recognize Your Thoughts and Feelings with Compassion

During the weeks and months following my painful losses, tending to my heart was a daily practice. I checked in with myself in simple ways, as I would a loved one in despair. I made space to be with God, to tune in to my thoughts and feelings, and seek wisdom.

Are you willing to experiment? Would you like to find out what can happen when you pause, take a deep breath, and invite the Holy Spirit to gently explore your heart with you? You may be surprised by the goodness He reveals. Grace and love walk hand in hand with grief.[121]

An Invitation to Action

1. During the 15 to 30 minutes you've set aside for this healing work, use five of those minutes to tune into your emotions and build emotional awareness.

   It's better to consistently spend a few focused minutes, than to aim for more than you can realistically manage. The goal is to create a regular rhythm of meeting with God in a quiet, comfortable space free from distractions as much as possible.

2. Breathe on Purpose—Take a few minutes to breathe slowly and intentionally. Let your body settle and your mind move toward peace. Offer yourself—and everything you're going through—to God. Gently invite the Holy Spirit to search your heart and bring light to what's happening inside.

   To grow in emotional awareness, ask yourself these three questions:

   What am I feeling? - Identify three emotions you're experiencing. Use the *Feeling Chart* below to help you find the right words. Then, rate the intensity of each emotion on a scale from 1 to 10 (low to high). *If you can name it, you can tame it.*

   What triggered these emotions? - Write down what was happening, or what you were thinking about, when you noticed these feelings.

   What thoughts are connected to these feelings? - Describe the specific thoughts attached to the emotions. Reflect with compassion—consider any relevant "who, what, when, where, or why" details.

   Over time, look back through your journal. You'll begin to see clear signs of growth and healing written in your own words.

My Feelings

INTENSITY OF FEELINGS

HAPPY	SAD	ANGRY	SCARED	ASHAMED
Excited	Depressed	Furious	Terrified	Defamed
Overjoyed	Agonized	Enraged	Horrified	Remorseful
Elated	Alone	Outraged	Scared stiff	Dishonored
Thrilled	Hurt	Boiling	Fearful	Admonished
Fired Up	Sorrowful	Irate	Panicky	
	Miserable	Seething	Shocked	
Gratified	Heartbroken	Upset	Apprehensive	Apologetic
Cheerful	Somber	Mad	Frightened	Sneaky
Satisfied	Lost	Defended	Insecure	Guilty
Relieved	Distressed	Frustrated	Uneasy	Secretive
Glowing	Melancholy	Agitated	Intimidated	
	Let Down	Disgusted	Threatened	
Glad	Unhappy	Perturbed	Nervous	Ridiculous
Pleasant	Moody	Annoyed	Worried	Regretful
Tender	Blue	Uptight	Timid	Pitied
Pleased	Upset	Irritated	Unsure	Silly
Mellow	Disappointed	Touchy	Anxious	
	Dissatisfied	Resistant	Cautious	

© 2017 The Empty Arms Journal

© PAM VREDEVELT | PAMVREDEVELT.COM | VREDEVELT MINISTRIES

If you can name it, you can tame it.

3. Watch Out for Unhealthy Thought Patterns - These three questions can help you spot mental habits that may be keeping you stuck in pain longer than necessary:

    - What negative thoughts or emotions keep looping in my mind? Consider thoughts and feeling connected with fear, anger, guilt, regret, or shame. Write them down.

    - Have I been replaying toxic thoughts? This might include ideas around blame, revenge, "would've/could've/should've," "what ifs," "if onlys," or hopeless thinking. Take a moment to jot down what you've noticed.

    - Where has my mind been drifting on auto-pilot? Make a quick note of where your thoughts tend to drift when you aren't focused on something.

4. Write Yourself a Compassion Letter – With kindness and love thank your heart, soul, mind, and body for how they've carried you through the pain of your losses. Acknowledge how each part of you has endured deep heartache and helped you keep going. If you've been hard on yourself, offer an apology. Forgive yourself for anything you're holding against yourself.

    Then, describe three specific ways you will show yourself more compassion and silence self-criticism going forward. These might be small daily actions, kind thoughts, or simple practices that remind you you're worthy of care.[122]

Notice your focus. What you focus on grows and influences your quality of life.

Don't be discouraged when unexpected things arise and disrupt your time with God. Life is full of interruptions—and that's okay. When plans get thrown off, it doesn't mean you've failed. Just begin again as soon as you can.

Give yourself grace, and hold your heart gently in a space free from judgment.[123] Be honest with God, and with yourself, about what's real. He's not keeping score—He simply longs to be with you.

What matters most is that you continue to come back, keep connecting with God and making time to mend.[124] One moment at a time, one breath at a time—you're healing, and He's with you in every step.

Remember, your grief is as unique as your fingerprint—no one else experiences it quite the way you do. It's shaped by your love, your story, and your loss. So please, be gentle with yourself.

Offer your heart the kindness it needs to heal. Give yourself full permission to listen—really listen—to what your soul is saying. Allow your emotions to speak without a hint of judgment and meet them with compassion.

Keep your approach simple:

"*Recognize* what your heart is saying with compassion."

Can you imagine those words glowing, like warm neon light in the dark? Let the image settle into your memory—a gentle reminder to treat yourself with the same grace you would offer a friend you love.

Healing isn't to be rushed. Just honored. One tender step at a time.

In God's economy, transformation rhythms are gradual and gentle. Guidance is wisely paced. God knows you better than you know yourself, is fully aware of your needs, and will provide in ways unknown to you.

In the safety of God's love, stay open and watch for what unfolds. God will meet you there. And little by little, you'll begin to notice quiet glimmers of freedom rising within you—subtle, beautiful signs that healing is happening.[125]

This is how mending works: not all at once, but one careful stitch at a time.

People from every background have walked this path, choosing to partner with God in the slow, sacred work of healing their hearts.[126] Many still carry the rewards today—a deeper sense of peace, renewed purpose, and the joy of becoming a lifeline for others in pain. Their flourishing wasn't accidental. They made the choice to show up and keep practicing.

They discovered something true: *practice doesn't make perfect—practice makes better.*

You can do the same. You can learn, grow, and confidently partner with God—not only to mend your own heartheartbeak, but also to bring comfort and hope to others.

Count on this: every small act of care adds up. Each gentle step forward invites more grace, more strength, and more faith for what lies ahead.

The greater your pain, the greater God's provision. The bigger your need, the bigger the opportunity to trust God's regenerating power that, at this very moment, is mightily working *in* you.[127]

Amazing mysteries are yet to be revealed along your path of becoming new.

10

ANGEL VISITS IN THE DARK

Believers, look up—take courage.
The angels are nearer than you think.

Billy Graham

The next few pages you are about to read are difficult for me to openly share. They detail my most vulnerable raw moments of grief, which honestly, I'd prefer to privately tuck away and not expose.

So, why do I bother telling this part of my story? First, because I'm committed to the HOW (being Honest, Open, and Willing) in my connection with you. Secondly, I'd like to shine a glimmer of light into the dense fog of your grief, and gently draw attention to the supernatural realm that surrounds each one of us. Triune Love and angels on assignment are always close to us, whether we recognize them or not.[128] Allow me a little room to explain what I mean.

* * *

Sirens screamed through the air. Red lights flashed in every direction, like a disco ball lighting up the night sky.

"Oh God!" Jessie cried. "Please, NO, not..."

Sprinting barefoot across the street, our daughter, Jessie, pried her way through a long row of bushes, searching for a place in the fence to see what was happening. Waving her arms wildly and shouting at the top of her voice, she tried to catch the police officers' attention. It was no use. They couldn't hear her over the freeway noise.

Just then, our friend, Caroleena, noticed Jessie by the fence and guided an officer over to her.

4 Hours Earlier...

Our family had been invited to join our friends in their suite for a Portland Trail Blazers basketball game. Nathan loved watching the Blazers play ball!

John came down with a feverish flu that morning, so Matt and Caroleena used our tickets to take Nathan to the game. Matt, an experienced special education assistant, knew Nathan well. He was his big buddy (a.k.a. personal aid) at summer camp and Nathan thought he was so cool.

The second-quarter clock ticked down to zero, the arena buzzing with excitement. The Portland Trail Blazers were giving the San Antonio Spurs a thorough licking. Jessie and Nathan enjoyed the terrific fun while sharing a sandwich and soda.

During half-time, Jessie leaned over to Nathan, tapped the side of her face with her finger, and asked for a kiss. Every now and then, she got lucky, and Nathan gave her a quick peck on the cheek. This time, Nathan blushed with embarrassment, shyly retreated, and waved her away saying, "Ahhhhh...No...."

"Well, then can I give you a kiss?" Jessie asked.

"Ahhhh....O-tay," Nathan said, squeamishly giving in.

Jessie planted a big red smooch on his cheek, which he promptly wiped off with a grin.

Jessie invited Nathan to use the bathroom inside the suite before the second half started. He lined up behind several others, agreeing to patiently wait his turn.

Jessie's fiancé, Chris, checked on Nathan a few minutes later. The line had dwindled and the bathroom door was locked. Chris knocked but all was quiet. Nathan didn't like interruptions and often didn't answer anyone when he was in the bathroom. Chris figured Nathan wanted privacy and waited in the wings. He understood the idiosyncrasies of children with special needs having grown up with an adopted sister who was developmentally delayed.

Just then, Caroleena's husband, Matt burst into the suite and collapsed to the floor, struggling for air. He barely managed to choke out the words, "Nathan was hit by a car outside the Moda Center."

With a backbone of steel and fiery focus, Jessie replied, "Matt, this is no time to fall apart. Pull yourself together. We have to get to Nathan!"

Jessie and Chris ran full speed outside for more information. A police officer told them Nathan was conscious when the ambulance left for Emanuel Hospital. Chris drove while Jessie pulled out her phone. Gathering her wits with a deep breath, she dialed my number and waited.

"Mom... are you sitting down?" she asked.

My stomach tied in knots hearing her tone of voice. Something was obviously wrong.

"Mom, Nathan was hit by a car. He's in an ambulance on the way to Emanuel Hospital. Can you meet us there?"

Adrenaline surged through my body. With my heart pounding fiercely in my chest, I wanted to hide and rage all at the same time. I flew through the kitchen gathering my things, giving John the news, and digging frantically in my purse for the car keys.

My phone rang again.

"Hello, I'm calling from Emanuel Hospital. Is this Mrs. Vredevelt?"

"Yes, it is," my voice quivered.

"Your son is here with us. He was hit by a car and the trauma doctors are with him now. Can you come to Emanuel Hospital Emergency?"

"Yes, of course!"

"Do you have someone who can drive you?"

"No! My husband is sick with the flu. I'm coming now!"

Pressing the accelerator to the floor, I cried, "Oh God, please be merciful to Nathan."

It was a request I had prayed many times for our boy. Growing up with special needs wasn't easy for him.

Intrusive images of Nathan being hit by a car triggered an explosive fury of emotion. Wave upon wave of nausea grew larger, demanding an exit.

"Breathe, Pam... breathe..."

I could barely see the road through swelling tears spilling down my face. Suddenly the traffic stopped cold, trapping me in a string of cars locked down for miles. Thousands of vehicles leaving the Trail Blazers game were motionless or barely creeping. I had no idea that Nathan's accident was causing the traffic jam.

Escaping the main road, I drove through a maze of side streets toward the hospital and hit one dead end after another. Powerlessness can bury you alive if you let it. I took several deep breaths, pulled to the curb, and called the hospital for directions.

A kind woman on the line talked me through the local streets into the hospital emergency lot. Jessie met me at the door and walked me into a busy lobby swarming with people.

My eyes fell instantly on Matt and Caroleena, the young couple who had taken Nathan to the game. Tears streamed down Matt's face as he apologized over and over again. Embracing them both, I tried every possible way to reassure them that the accident wasn't their fault. It could have happened on anyone's watch.

A short, dark-haired woman interrupted us. "The doctors need to talk with you, and then I'll take you to Nathan."

We entered a small conference room around the corner, where the trauma team introduced themselves and reviewed the facts.

"Nathan's legs and pelvis are broken. There are other internal injuries, but our biggest concern is his head trauma. His brain is swelling, and we need to act fast to relieve the pressure."

I could barely wrap my mind around what I was hearing. Without immediate surgery, Nathan would die. With surgery, the doctors didn't know if he would live.

I stood there suspended in disbelief. Just hours ago, Nathan and I were laughing and hugging one another. Now I was numb to the bone, robotically signing papers for doctors to save my son.

A heavy sinking feeling took over. Movement around me shifted into slow motion with hues of unreality. Panic swelled in my chest. My legs felt like there were hundred-pound weights strapped to my ankles walking the sterile hall toward Nathan.

We turned a corner into a small foyer. Glaring overhead fluorescents reflected off metal guardrails on both sides of Nathan lying motionless on a gurney.

"Oh, Nathan!" I screamed without making a sound.

Bloody gauze wrapped Nathan's head, partially covering bruises and pavement burns. Gently taking his hand, I leaned in close to speak in his ear, my tears falling on his cheek. I wanted him to feel my touch, hear my voice, and know I was with him.

"Hi, Nathan. I'm here now… Dad will be here soon. We're with you, buddy. I'm so sorry you are going through this. I love you, Nathan. I'm just… so… sorry."

Carefully cupping his face in my hand, I prayed, "Dear God, be with Nathan. Let him feel your love. Give the doctors wisdom. Help them take good care of my boy."

I wasn't sure my bones would hold me up if I let go of Nathan, but the surgeon kept pressing, "We have to move quickly."

Gently kissing his cheek I whispered one last time, "I love you, Nathan. I'll see you soon."

I watched the team wheel Nathan down the hall, until the eerie sound of double metal doors locked behind them.

Mary, a hospital social worker, walked me to a private waiting room.

My senses were inundated. Intellectually, I knew that Nathan was in critical condition, but emotionally I was drowning, swimming blind in my own skin. I needed to breathe, to slow the trembling vibrations threatening a meltdown.

Sinking into the chair, I leaned my head back against the cushion and closed my eyes. The room was quiet. My hands were cold. Mary said my face was as pale as the walls.

John drove immediately to wait with Jessie and me through Nathan's surgery. Several friends came and stayed by our side.

We were flailing in uncharted territory. The night watch had only begun.

***

A close friend walked over to us and knelt down in front of John and me. Charonne is a woman of continual prayer who clings to God like a vine on a trellis. In the forty years we've known her, we've admired her intelligence and keen sensitivity to God and people. A well-respected wife, mother, and retired school principal, Charonne is one of the most discerning individuals we've ever known.

Char and her husband, Al, knew what it was like to have a child teetering on the edge of life and death. Their fourteen-year-old son, Dustin, suffered severe brain injuries in a skateboarding accident. They walked with Dustin through grueling years of recovery and spent long stints travailing on their knees.

Today Dustin is a manager at one of the world's largest and most advanced semiconductor companies. The doctors say his healing is nothing short of miraculous.

Charonne's piercing blue eyes met mine, and I sensed a nudge alerting me to pay close attention.

"Pam and John, I see an angel standing at the head of Nathan's bed. He's intent, watching Nathan closely. It's the same angel that Nathan saw behind his rocking chair when he was little. He's massive and strong. I don't know what all this means, but I'm certain of one thing, Nathan is not alone."

Tears welled in my eyes as I wondered about the role of Nathan's sacred messenger. Was the angel dispatched to communicate something important to Nathan? Did it come to assist the doctors? Was this a guardian on assignment to escort Nathan to heaven?

My mind drifted back to all the evenings I spent alone with Nathan in the rocking chair. I hadn't thought about *that* angel in a very long time.

From the day we brought him home after he was born, Nathan and I had a bedtime routine. We nestled together in a big stuffed rocking chair, and I sang songs while rocking him. He lay in my arms, his eyes fixed on mine, until the picture blurred and he drifted off to sleep.

One night when Nathan was eighteen months old, I was feeding him at bedtime. But rather than looking at me—as he had every other night—he kept turning his head toward the blank wall on the opposite side of the nursery. It was dark, and for the life of me, I couldn't see anything there to distract him and hold his attention.

Each time he turned away his mouth lost suction, and milk ran down his cheek onto me. Wanting to fill his belly for the night and keep my pants dry, I tried turning his head back toward me for the fourth time. It was no use.

His sights were locked onto something on that wall. But there was nothing there. No shadows, no pattern of light. Nothing.

I was curious and softly asked, "Nathan, what are you looking at? What do you see?"

Dumb question. Even if he had been able to talk (which was not yet within his ability), his mouth was plugged drinking! For some unknown reason, I asked, "Nathan, do you see angels?"

I still don't know why I asked that question because angels weren't a common topic of conversation in our home. We didn't have children's books about angels, so the concept would have been completely foreign to Nathan. But when I said the word *angel*, it seemed obvious that Nathan understood.

He riveted his attention back on the blank wall and smiled from ear to ear! It was as if he were saying, "Way to go, Mom. You finally got it!"

I hid that incident in my heart and nearly forgot about it until Nathan was three years old. The scene was much the same. The same rocker. The same time of evening. The same nightly routine. But rather than lying in my arms, this time he tucked his little knees up on my lap and snuggled in, resting his head on my shoulder while I sang.

We were both nearly asleep, when all of us sudden he bolted straight back, bounced up and down, and pointed wildly behind the rocker, shouting "Aaa! Aaa! Aaa!" I was very tired that night and just wanted to crawl in bed for the night. Impatient with his antics I said, "Nathan, it is not time to play. It's time to go to sleep!"

But he kept bouncing, pointing behind the chair, and shouting, "Aaa! Aaa! Aaa!" His persistence triggered the memory of an earlier time when he'd stared and smiled at the dark blank wall.

"Nathan," I asked, "Do you see angels?"

This time he said, "Da!" with a smile. Content with my acknowledgment, he put his head back down on my shoulder and promptly fell asleep. "Da" is "Yes" in Nathan's vocabulary.

Still somewhat skeptical, I ran a test the next morning. When our friend, Margaret, came to the house, I said, "Nathan, can you show Margaret where you saw the angels last night?"

He took her by the hand, marched her into the nursery, and pointed behind the rocking chair.

My previous doubts vanished that day.

Footsteps in the hall interrupted my musings.

Nathan's doctors had an update: "We removed a small portion of Nathan's skull to give his brain room to swell. It's too early to tell whether or not he will survive. It's a waiting game now. We need to watch his brain over the next few days. In the meantime, we're doing everything possible to keep him comfortable."

I pressed to know more: "Nathan adores his big brother, Ben, who is at college in Nashville, Tennessee. Do we need to fly Ben home?"

Studying the doctor's faces, I searched for clues with no success. Their answers were vague and elusive for good reason. There were too many unknowns to make predictions.

Mary, the social worker, stood close. When the doctors headed back to the surgical center, the fearless conviction in Mary's eyes spoke louder than her words, "I suggest you get Nathan's brother on the first plane out of Nashville."

Jessie and I took the elevator to the Pediatric Intensive Care Unit where Nathan would be taken after surgery. John couldn't risk exposing others to the flu, so he went home. It was late. We were exhausted and dazed by the day's trauma.

Jessie refused to leave, determined to stay the night with Nathan in his room. The kind nurses on duty didn't disturb her when she crawled into bed next to Nathan. Gently stroking his skin, she whispered prayers over him through the night.

My thoughts darted in every direction trying to make sense of things, but the search for logic only ended in knee-buckling overwhelm. I could not fathom life without Nathan.

Hoping to salvage some semblance of sanity before dawn, I followed John home to rest.

Little did we know that sacred mysteries awaited us. In the hushed hours of the night, heaven touched earth.

An Invitation to Action

1. Write in your journal about a time when you, or someone you know, wondered if angels were involved in the situation.

2. Explore Your Reactions to the Unexplainable: How do you typically respond when something mysterious or unexplainable happens? What thoughts or emotions come up? What do you believe about supernatural encounters, and how did you come to those beliefs?

3. Describe a time when you—or someone you know—experienced something mysterious, miraculous, or clearly guided by God, that seemed beyond human explanation.

4. Seek God's Perspective: Ask God what He wants you to understand about the experiences you described in #1 and #3. Spend a few quiet moments listening, and write down what comes to mind.

11

GOD ENCOUNTERS

*If we find ourselves with a desire that nothing in this
world can satisfy, the most probable explanation
is that we were made for another world.*
C.S. Lewis

I crawled into bed seeking comfort in John's embrace. Shutting off the chatter racing in my mind was next to impossible. Ever so slowly, sleep descended providing a hint of escape from the brutal realities.

During the wee hours of the morning, I rolled over, pulled the covers around my chin, and squinted at just the right time to see the clock tic 3:00 a.m. In one earth-stopping transcendent moment, I heard a whisper, "I'm going to bring him home."

God's kind-hearted presence was palpable. I don't know if my ears picked up the message audibly, or if it was discerned some other way. What I do know is that God was talking about Nathan.

I'm going to bring him home. Love's caring, gentle voice is forever etched in my memory.

We were being redirected. The intention conveyed was contrary to how we and thousands of people were praying across the country. Our family and friends were asking God to touch Nathan's broken body and heal him.

For years, we had the privilege of seeing miracles up close—praying with people both here and around the world. In so many places, especially in third-world countries, we saw how the childlike faith of those we served made room for God to move powerfully. We saw tumors disappear, blind eyes see, backs straighten, heavy oppression lift, and diseases vanish.

When we prayed for Nathan, we came with that same expectant faith—believing for a miracle.

God heard our petitions and with great compassion entered our suffering to calm our hearts and unveil His plan.

The next morning, I told John about what I heard, second-guessing myself as I told the story.

"I think I heard God say, 'I'm going to bring him home.' I might be wrong. I was half asleep. Everything feels foggy and upside down…"

Gently squeezing my hand, John's reassurance interrupted me, "No, Pam," he said shaking his head, "When you hear, you hear."

Waves of indescribable sadness washed over us, sensing that our time with Nathan was quickly coming to an end.

On our way to the hospital, we called my parents in California.

Dad answered, relieved to hear our voices. He'd been waiting for our call.

From the moment Grandpa had laid eyes on Nathan, the two shared a unique bond. I have vivid memories of Dad holding Nathan as a baby in his favorite recliner, with tears of compassion rolling down his cheeks. He sensed the long rough road ahead of Nathan. Mom and Dad prayed every day for him and the rest of us.

"Dad, the doctors say that we're in wait-and-see mode for the next three days," I explained. "There are too many unknowns for them to predict an outcome. They say they've seen individuals with worse injuries survive, and others who were less injured not make it. They keep telling us they're holding out hope for Nathan to recover."

I told Dad about my 3:00 a.m. encounter, "I sense that God is going to take Nathan home."

"Honey, I do, too," he replied.

John glanced at me with a look on his face that said, "Did he just say what I think he said?!" Dad's instant agreement startled both of us. It was completely uncharacteristic for Dad to quickly conclude anything before carefully investigating and weighing all the details. Dad is a math genius who graduated with an Engineering degree from the U.S. Naval Academy. He's a deeply compassionate man of faith, a critical thinker, and a brilliant leader.

I silently wondered what drove his response. More of the story unfolded.

"I had trouble sleeping last night," he said. "Around 3:00 a.m., I got out of bed and went to the den to rest in my recliner. Mom was asleep, and the house was quiet. I threw a blanket over me, leaned back in my chair, and began praying for Nathan and all of you.

"I don't think I have the right words to explain what happened. It was like I was in a *zone*. I don't know if God gives us a chance to say goodbye to loved ones on our way to heaven, but at that moment, I somehow sensed Nathan was with me. He wanted me to know he was okay and that he loved me. Honey, I don't understand it all, but I know in my heart that Nathan is alright, and everything is going to be okay."

Dad's story left John and me speechless. We had never heard him talk like this before.

I marveled at the meticulous staging of these two 3:00 am encounters.[129] Seven hundred miles apart, at precisely the same moment, God said to me, "I'm going to bring him home," while Dad sensed Nathan's loving goodbye.

Overnight, it seemed, we suddenly became beholders of secret riches, priceless treasure mercifully given for love's sake.[130] Unbeknownst to us, heaven's gracious gifts, dispensed for the good of all, had only just begun.[131]

> *I will give you the treasures of darkness and hidden riches of secret places, that you may know that it is I, the Lord…Who calls you by your name.*
> *Isaiah 45:3, AMP*

Jessie's Vision (*as told by Jessie shortly after Nathan's accident*)

My little brother, Nathan, lay in a coma, on full life support in the pediatric ICU at Emmanuel Hospital. The day before, a car barreling 55 mph down the freeway hit him full force. The devastating impact caused a brain injury, broken bones, and other vital organ damage.

Our family took turns staying with Nathan around the clock. We held his hand, stroked his arms, sang of God's love, and spoke to Nathan about his priceless value.

We were tangled up in a bizarre twist of events. One minute, we were together at the Moda Center, cheering for our hometown basketball team, the Portland Trail Blazers. The next we were rallying people to search the arena for Nathan.

While waiting in line to use the suite restroom, Nathan quietly slipped out an adjacent door into a crowded foyer, bustling with half-time spectators searching for food and restrooms.

Nathan wasn't able to forecast unintended consequences, which I suppose, was both a blessing and a curse. He was born with Down syndrome and had a thing for bold adventure.

When Mom and Dad arrived at Nathan's room, I went to rest in an RV left for us by friends in the hospital parking lot. Curled up under a blanket on the bed, scenes of Nathan running through the dark onto the freeway, disoriented by lights speeding toward him, replayed over and over in my mind. I didn't want to close my eyes, for fear I'd relive the never-ending horror in my dreams. The torment of Nathan being alone, scared, and in horrible pain, was more than I could bear.

Just then, it was as if God pulled back a curtain and opened my eyes to see into the invisible realm. I was at the accident scene looking toward the rear of the ambulance, surrounded by black night. Paramedics were on the pavement working to revive Nathan. Light streamed into the darkness through the open doors of the empty ambulance.

And there was Nathan, sitting atop the back of the ambulance with Jesus, playfully kicking their legs back and forth, like kids on the end of a dock during a summer vacation. Nathan was beaming! Jesus had his arm around Nathan. They exchanged looks with each other like giddy best friends who hadn't been together for years.

The scene shifted to a close-up of Nathan. He looked like my little brother, but there was no trace of Down syndrome. He was radiant, whole, and thrilled to be with Jesus.

A twinkle in Nathan's eye and his playful grin said, "I've got a secret, Nana (his nickname for me). I know something you don't know. Ha-Ha!" There's no question in my mind that what I sensed was undeniably Nathan! He loved to tease me.

Jesus and Nathan watched the EMTs carefully recover his body from the ground and place it in the ambulance. Then as quickly as the picture emerged, it disappeared in a flash. I felt a sudden warm peace envelope me and I knew without a doubt, Nathan wasn't scared. He wasn't in pain, and Nathan definitely wasn't alone. Afterward, my mind didn't repaint Nathan's accident in flashback form ever again.

Our family calls it a mending miracle.

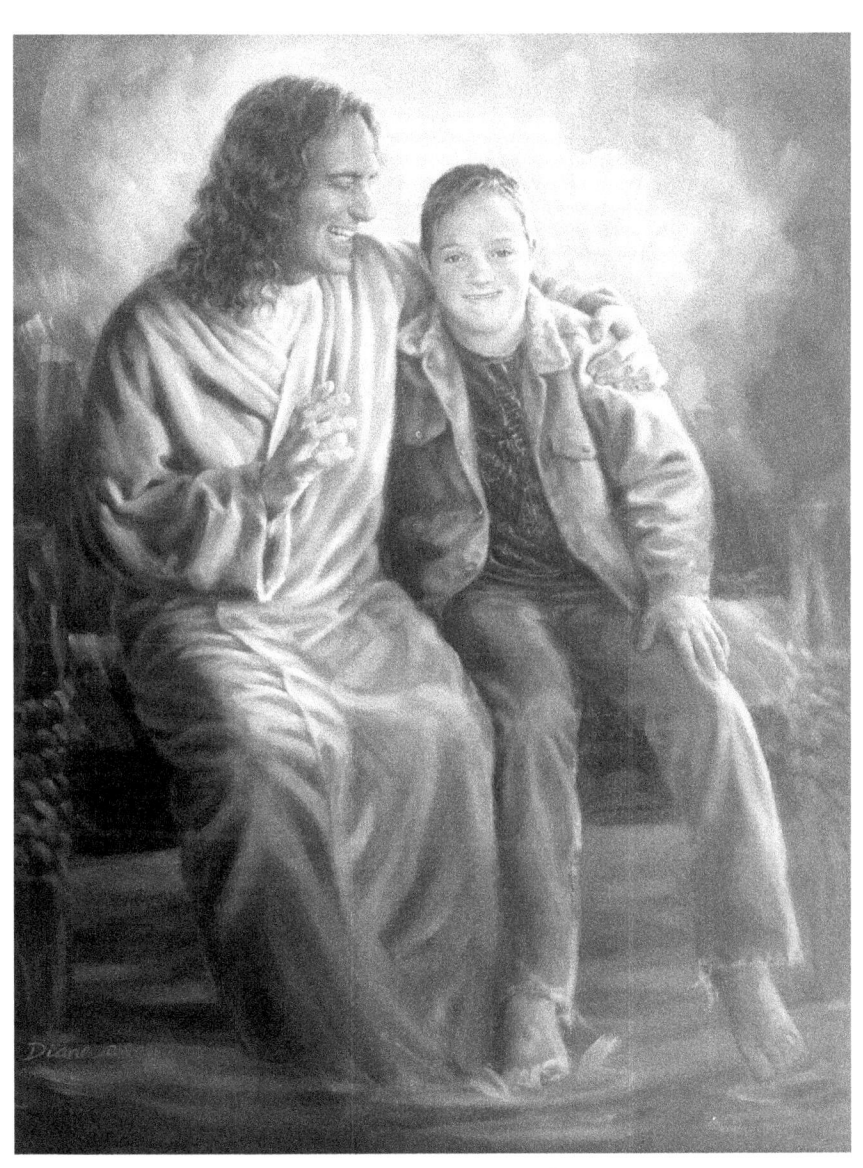

An Invitation to Action

1. Describe a time when you sensed a God whisper in your journal. What was the message, and how did you respond? Describe the thoughts and feelings you had at the time.

2. Describe how you typically pray for yourself and others who are hurting. When and how did you learn that approach?

3. Write an emotionally honest prayer in your journal:

    - Share with God what you want to experience more and less of during prayer.

    - Explain how unanswered prayers influence your current prayer practice.

    - Describe what you tend to conclude about God, about prayer, and about yourself when your prayers aren't answered the way you want.

    - Tell God your honest thoughts, feelings, and questions about spiritual encounters such as those described in the last two chapters.

12

TEAR TRACKINGS

A wounded heart will heal in time, and when it does, the memory and love of our lost ones is sealed inside to comfort us.

Brian Jacques

From the time he was a toddler, Nathan had a hard time grasping the fact that the boundaries we set in place were there for his protection. But in all fairness, I can't fault him. His special needs made learning more difficult. I also think he came by his drive for independence quite naturally. Don't most of us share this predisposition at the core of our humanity?

When we wander, don't we tend to forget a fundamental truth: God gives us boundaries to keep the good in and the bad out. Safety limits are for our protection.

God knows that when we separate ourselves and wander away from love, we end up confused and disoriented. We suffer. We lose quality of life. Relationships fly apart. We end up scared and broken. Part of our soul dies.

And Perfect Love looks on, wanting so much more for us. God knows better than anyone what it's like to have kids who wander. Moses said, "For the LORD your God…has known your wanderings."[133] He knows what it's like to hear his children cry out in the dark when they don't know where they are or how they got there. He knows about the times we bolt for a new measure of freedom and wind up getting iced or burned.

God knows when we find ourselves standing in the middle of a situation—vulnerable, bare, and unprotected from the elements at large.

His eyes fill with tears, too.

When young David was on the run from jealous King Saul, he was forced to spend long months and *years* in hiding.

Always on the move from place to place, he haunted the lonely wilderness like a lost soul, sometimes taking refuge in the depths of a limestone cave. When the fear and anger intensified, his eyes turned toward heaven flowing with tears from a heart filled with grief. With sore knees on the hard damp rocks of a cavern floor, he reminded himself of this truth:

You've kept track of my every toss and turn through the sleepless nights, each tear entered in your ledger, each ache written in your book.[134]

David says each one of your tears is taken into account.

In the Hebrew language, the word used here reflects a picture of a vineyard keeper carefully watching for each drop squeezed from grapes by a wine press, as he creates a very costly wine. What that says to me is that God doesn't take our pain lightly. He isn't casual about our weeping. He isn't nonchalant about our suffering.

Each tear holds tremendous value.

John and I traveled to Cairo, Egypt a while back and learned about various artifacts found in Egyptian tombs. One item was called a lachrymatory, or "tear bottle." The custom in ancient times was for friends to take tear bottles with them when they visited those who were ill or in great distress. As tears ran down the cheeks of the sufferer, friends caught the tears in the bottle and then sealed and preserved them as a memorial of the event.

We live in a time and culture foreign to this practice. Most of us would prefer to *forget* the painful times of life. We'd rather honor our joys and give them more prominence in our minds than our sorrows. But David says God sees things differently. What we like to forget, God takes great care to remember.

What gave David the ability to endure years of oppression and severe hardship?

A simple truth: *God remembers*. He keeps track.

He remembers every sleepless night. He remembers every prayer, every groan, and every heartache too deep for words. God remembers. That single thought changed David's trembling fear-ridden words into a brand-new confident declaration.

Following that pivotal awareness, David says, "Fearless now, I trust in God.... God, you did everything you promised, and I'm thanking you with all my heart. You pulled me from the brink of death, my feet from the cliff edge of doom. Now I stroll at leisure with God in the sunlit fields of life."[135]

God isn't partial. What He did for David, He does for you and me. He remembers. When no one else knows we are suffering, God does. He is with us, sitting by our side, catching the tears that roll off our cheeks. No sorrow goes undetected.

> *Crying doesn't mean you're weak... Sometimes
> it's what you need to do to get strong again.*
>
> J.W. Lynne

In God's economy, all suffering can serve a significant eternal purpose. Tears *never* go unnoticed. They are carefully collected, sealed, and saved as a sacred reminder of your journey.

God also understands the moments when we pull away—when we hold back our tears, turn inward, and drift from the warmth of His love. And still, He doesn't let us go. He's the One who stirs a grandmother's prayers on our behalf, who places a caring friend in our path to gently lead us home. He's the One who waits at the window, watching with hope and longing, inviting us back inside, out of the cold, into His sheltering grace.

His guardrails are not punishment, but protection—lovingly placed to keep the good in and the harm out.

Maybe that's why Jesus told the story of the lost son with such tenderness.[136] Because our God is a compassionate Father who never stops longing for us, who treasures every prayer, gathers every tear, and celebrates with joy whenever we return to Him.

An Invitation to Action

1. What healthy boundaries or practices do you currently have in place that help keep you grounded in your true self, connected to God, and in healthy relationship with others?

2. Growing up, what early messages did you learn—directly or indirectly—about crying and expressing grief? How did your parents or caregivers model responses to loss?

3. What are two important things you've learned about grief that have helped you experience more freedom and healing?

4. Choose one trusted person to share these insights with. After your conversation, take a moment to reflect in your journal: What was it like to share these truths? What did you feel or notice during the experience?

13

LOVE TALKS

When you take your cues from the Holy Spirit, you'll do some things that will make people think you're crazy. So be it. Obey the whisper and see what God does.

Mark Batterson

"Hmmm... Partner with God to mend my broken heart? I guess I've never really thought about it. Are you talking about something different than asking God to heal me?" Haley said.

The honest question spilled from an open wound. Haley, a bright professional thirty-something, was at her wits' end after a very close friend and work associate unpredictably cut off all communication and refused to talk to her. Two months of this hostile silent treatment kicked Haley's confidence to the curb, leaving her grief-stricken, walking off-balance on eggshells.

"Haley, that's a great question!" I responded. "It's not an all-or-nothing, either/or situation. Think of it as a 'both/and,' like a team effort (**t** – together, **e** – everyone, **a** – achieves, **m** – more). You do your part, and God does His. It's a rich interactive process that's far more creative and collaborative than trying to heal your heart alone, or passively waiting for God to do it."

Haley was curious and eager to know more about how a healing *partnership* with God might work. I offered an explanation, similar to what I've shared with many in the counseling office:

The strategy comes from a pattern seen in the lives of people throughout history. Their case studies, documented in the best-selling book of all time, highlight long lists of traumatic incidents, scathing friendship betrayals, and tragic losses woven together with supernatural guidance, grace, and redemption. Their stories give us a window into the agonies they endured, the ways they experienced God, and their unstoppable resilience to rise up and transcend their losses with vibrancy and purpose.

The practices I'd like to suggest, offer life-changing opportunities. I say this because I know firsthand that they work. I've used them for decades and watched countless individuals in the counseling office benefit from them as well. Through these simple practices, you partner with God to mend your heart, and at the same time learn what an intimate friendship with God is meant to be. It's an experiential journey that gives plenty of room for individual initiative and creativity on your part and for customized healing guidance on God's part.

In the context of reliable, intelligible conversations with God, you address the tangled matters of your heart in Love's presence. Working together with God, you tend to your heart wounds little by little, addressing specific matters. Slowly but surely, you follow God's lead moving incrementally toward abundant wholeness.[137]

I showed Haley a picture of this portable, productive process that can be used anytime, anywhere. The four-part cycle provides a clear, practical way to develop an interactive friendship with God, within which you partner to mend your broken heart. The model offers two gifts:

- a clear plan that guides and guards you from pitfalls on your healing journey

- a toolbox with vocabulary, words, images, and practices that promote healing and renewal on your way *through* grief.

The framework is my concerted effort to blend together insights from my fifty-year friendship with God, the timeless wisdom of God's love letters, robust clinical research, and forty years of private practice as a therapist. It's my attempt to integrate concepts from theology, psychology, neurobiology, and grief science to offer sound practices for emotional healing in companionship with God.

Within the paradigm, I clarify what I understand as God's part and our part in the healing journey. It's not Gospel carved in stone, but it is good news that potentially holds timeless benefits for you, your loved ones, and the generations that follow.

Let me pull back the lens and offer a bird's eye view of the framework I call Love Talks:

LOVE TALKS

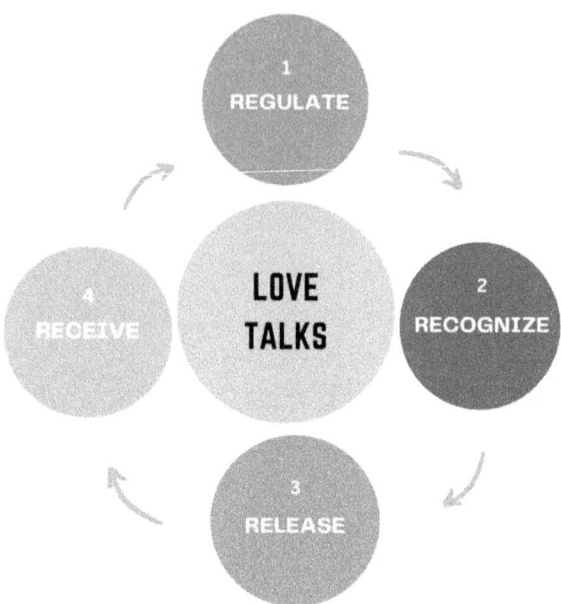

We'll take a close look at each of the four elements in the Love Talk cycle, and you'll learn step-by-step how to use it. My goal in sharing this framework is to invite you into an effective practice to confidently mend your emotional wounds in the context of your friendship with God and others. The Wonderful Counselor, who lives *within* you, will lead the way and orchestrate your transformation experience through grief into abundant wholeness.[138][139]

When you intentionally bring your grief into the light of Triune Love (your part), you can count on God's all-knowing presence to illuminate and guide your awareness in specific ways that foster understanding, growth, and freedom for your particular life situation (God's part).[140][141]

Love Talks are a natural, central part of building your friendship with God and key to restoring your peace and purpose. If these ideas are new to you, I encourage you to approach them with curiosity. Stay **H**onest, **O**pen, and

Willing to explore the options and possibilities. You are completely free to decide what you do with the insights you gain.

The Love Talk process begins at the top of the cycle with *Regulate*. In Chapter 5 you learned a variety of ways to reset and regulate your heart-soul-mind-body. You practiced using the power of breathing on purpose (B.O.P.) to exchange a noisy pounding pace, for the peaceful quiet calm in God's presence.

In stillness with God, the next step is to *Recognize* your inner world (thoughts, feelings, conflicts) with compassion — the same compassion you would demonstrate toward a good friend. Embraced in God's love, you curiously search your heart with the Holy Spirit. While intentionally turning toward your heartache, you gently identify and acknowledge your thoughts and feelings in a no-judgment zone, knowing that whatever is revealed can be healed. You already have this skill in your toolbox after implementing the action steps in Chapter 9.

Then you move on to *Release* your grief, those messy thoughts and feelings that rise to the surface while exploring your inner world with the Holy Spirit. You let go of painful e-motion (energy in motion) along with whatever thoughts are attached to those feelings while talking with God. After releasing your current burden to love, you open your heart to *Receive* intimate expressions of God's goodness. God exchanges your heartache with His grace gifts, custom fit to meet your needs at the time. This process of releasing and receiving is explained in detail in Chapter 14.

It can help to see real-life examples of everyday people, similar to you and me, who have used these practices in partnership with God to mend and flourish after devastating losses. I'll introduce you to a number of people, but first I'd like you to meet one of my role models, David, the second ruler of the united kingdom of ancient Israel and Judah.

As a famous world influencer, he was most well-known for his strengths, but he repeatedly encountered God through the humble admission of his vulnerabilities, weaknesses, and flaws. That's the part of him that resonates most with me and inspires me to grow.

The ways he partnered with God through a lifetime of unthinkable tragedies and resiliently prevailed, are second to none. Why? He did his part. He earnestly sought God with an **H**onest, **O**pen, and **W**illing heart. God was always available, just as he is for you and me, to meet him in his pain, to exchange his grief with good gifts, and ultimately to redeem his losses.[142]

Did you know God is always ready, waiting at the door of your heart, eager to meet with you, too?[143] He will never stop patiently knocking, because Love is passionate about making you whole, and free.

A beautiful friend, 91 years young, recently lost her husband and shared with me the story of her very first Love Talk. One simple question and one clear answer broke through unrelenting worries, and lifted her into a place of peace.[144]

My husband of 23 years passed away after a long hard struggle with Parkinson's. I was conflicted by numerous self-doubts over how I grieved his absence.

My grief looked different from what my friends experienced after their own heartbreaking losses. I missed my husband terribly, but I was very calm and relieved for him that his suffering was over.

He was at peace. I never doubted for a moment that Dave was in heaven or that I would see him again.

A good friend, who also happens to be a therapist, suggested I talk with God about what was bothering me. I had never tried having a two-way conversation with God before, so this was a new experience.

One evening I sat quietly alone in my living room and simply asked God to speak to me. I asked Him to tell me if I was doing what He wished, or if what I was doing was at least passable. In the comfortable stillness I waited.

Almost immediately the answer came, "It's okay. I've been there, too." Instant relief washed over me. I was freed of worry and concern.

I'm confident that God spoke because that answer would never occur to me. To this day, I'm not fully certain of what was meant by, 'I've been there, too.' Maybe Jesus was reassuring me that He, too, wrestled with self-doubt within His own experience of being fully human.

If I asked my therapist friend, she'd encourage me to seek God for more understanding. But right now, I'm content knowing that I'm okay. I feel loved, appreciated and safe. It's a really good feeling.

LOVE TALK   *Marilyn - age 91*

An Invitation to Action

1. Take a picture of the Love Talks diagram, print it out, and stick it on your refrigerator. Whenever you open the fridge for food or a drink, rehearse the four R's: Regulate, Recognize with Compassion, Release, and Receive. Love Talks is such a simple practice that even children can use it to become more aware of their thoughts and feelings in their daily conversations with God.

2. As you read the next chapter, Hearing Matters, place a star in the margin next to any thoughts, emotions, and questions you want to bring up in conversation with God.

14

HEARING MATTERS

Remember, you are held safe. You are loved. You are protected. You are in communion with God and with those whom God has sent you. What is of God will last. It belongs to the eternal life. Choose it, and it will be yours.

Henry Nouwen

He was the tall, lanky guy in seventh grade with pretty eyes, who knew just what to say to pull you out of the dumps. Most people didn't pay much attention to him back then. He was sort of a loner, usually off by himself scribbling notes or making music for an audience of one. Yet, during his awkward adolescent years, this reflective solitary teen was chosen over seven smart strapping older brothers to rule the United Kingdom of

Israel.[145] What launched this young unknown outsider to the front of the dynasty line?

One strength seems to stand out above all others. David is the only person in recorded history who God identified as "a man after God's own heart."[146]

Do you know that David is mentioned over 600 times in the Bible? 66 chapters in the Old Testament speak of David. He's mentioned fifty-nine times in the New Testament. The intimacies of David's heart spilled into seventy-three poetic songs before 1000 BC, continue to resonate with men and women around the globe to this day.

78 percent of the Psalms are songs of lament. These multi-dimensional portraits of David show him truthfully baring his soul to God in grave despair. More is written in the Bible about David's hopes and fears, emotional suffering, and personal transformation than any other human being.

Historians agree that few individuals in Scripture have had as much influence on later traditions as David. His story is told against the backdrop of the monarchy of the newly united tribes of Israel in the tenth century BC, and his life served as a model for national rulers through multiple generations.[147] David was far from perfect, but his passionate faith made him the model Israel's future kings tried to follow.

His path from the sheep pastures of childhood to the royal palace was long and arduous, strewn with physical and emotional carnage. David knew well the heartrending impact of loss and trauma.[148] Like most of us, there were moments when David buckled under the weight of unrelenting grief and the mental torment of fierce gloom and regret. Anxieties nagged him through lonely nights, as he tossed and turned staring into dark unknowns, restlessly waiting for the dawn.[149]

Psalm 27 describes one of many troubling times in David's life when everyone and everything he loves is gone. His plans are shattered. He's vulnerable, on the run, hiding in an alien place. His friends walk out and evil closes in. Personal and national threats loom on the horizon.

From the depths of aching loneliness, in a place of never-ending deadness as far as the eye can see, David rallies all his affection toward one direction and cries: "The one thing I want from God, the thing I seek most of all, is the privilege of meditating in his Temple, living in his presence every day of my life, delighting in his incomparable perfections and glory."[150]

A picture emerges. We see a single-minded person desperate for one thing—he wanted God to fill his aching void. David chose to daily pursue companionship with God, to experientially know His heart and mind. Quickly responding to God's voice was his default way of life.

> *My heart has heard you say, "Come and talk with me."*
> *And my heart responds, "Lord, I am coming."* [151]

What allowed David to maintain his childlike curiosity, wonder, and spontaneous delight while enduring life-altering, worst-case scenarios? What empowered David to persevere and ascend to elevated heights of faith and influence, against outlandishly cruel odds stacked against him?

History is clear. David's intimate friendship with God was key. David wasn't content to simply know *about* God from an intellectual distance. He passionately wanted to know God firsthand. With a heart of faith, on both good days and bad, David practiced shifting his attention to God to talk about what was on his mind.

Communing in Love's presence was a daily act of David's will, a routine of sorts, which eventually flamed into fervent desire. This one intentional practice (or the absence of it) led to significant life-changing outcomes for David, as well as for all those within his circle of influence.[152]

In seasons of deep mourning, David sought wisdom from God—who always speaks in love, without reproach or condemnation. Jamie Winship, world-renowned thought leader and co-founder of Identity Exchange, highlights two distinct patterns in David's life and their outcomes:

- **David thought to himself** – relying solely on human reasoning led David to operate out of a false identity, which resulted in defeat.

- **David inquired of the Lord** – engaging in honest conversation with God, David stepped into his true identity, followed divine wisdom, and experienced victory.[153]

These clear patterns are seen throughout his story. When David listened and responded to God's voice, in spite of any push-back received from others, he thrived.[154] On the other hand, when David thought to himself,[155] making decisions without consulting God, his problems multiplied and produced painful results.[156]

David wasn't perfect. He was a person like you and me, whose human frailty, pride, and tendency to pull away from God led to major blunders. However, in the overall scheme of things, David's typical disciplined practice was to pursue God in conversation.[157] And when his missteps were brought to light, David acknowledged the truth, did an about-face in his thinking, and humbly sought forgiveness.[158]

David didn't run from God in his pain and suffering. Even when he brought misery upon himself through poor judgment and blatant wrong-doing, David still turned around and ran *to* God. His example of contrite truth-telling invites the rest of us *imperfects* to seek God's help with our own heart wounds, self-inflicted or not.[159]

I imagine David honed the skill of lifting his eyes to heaven and tuning in to his Maker as a young boy, while tending his father's sheep in wide-open places. Over the years, those quiet moments became his training ground. God became his closest confidant—his secret place—right there in the open fields around Bethlehem. His song mirrors his practice: "He who dwells in the secret place of the Most High shall abide under the shadow of the Almighty. I will say of the LORD, 'He is my refuge and my fortress; my God, in Him I will trust.'"[160] In the presence of Triune Love, David safely released his burdens and received relief beyond what this world offers. He lingered long with his closest friend, off-loading irrational fears, confusion, and lonely longings, making space for love to mend and restore.

During the activities of the day and silence of the night, David developed his listening skills through regular practice. He didn't make tuning into God complicated. He simply found a comfortable place, took off his shoes, relaxed, and focused his mind on God.

External distractions under the sky overhead were mostly limited to chirping birds, wind whistling through trees, and occasional bleating lambs. David didn't have to shut out the noisy technostress[161] of today's world that steals healthy brain development[162] and contentment from those of us carrying smartphones.[163] [164]

At the end of the day when all was still, I wonder if David struggled to quiet the ceaseless chatter of his inner critic, like you and I do.

We don't have all the answers. But what we do know is that David didn't hide his hurt or his questions. He kept his heart open to the One who loved him unconditionally and knew every detail of his life. David truly wanted to bring joy to God, not sadness, so he regularly surrendered everything—his will, his thoughts, instincts, senses, and emotions. He invited the Light to search his heart and magnify whatever needed attention, while trusting the Master Mender to care for his heart.[165] [166]

David's conversations with God are often described like a movie running through his mind. He asked questions and listened for God's perspective. He paid close attention and carefully described in writing the words, pictures, images, feelings, and impressions he experienced while talking with Love.

No question was too small or too silly to ask. No cry of his heart was too angry, too offensive, or too shameful to bring into the Light. He knew any topic was safe with God. Somewhere along the way, David learned *whatever is revealed can be healed.*

Allow me to add a side note here: *Whatever God reveals, is intended to heal.* The Holy Spirit is the kindest person you'll ever meet. He doesn't disclose the truth to embarrass or humiliate you.[167] God always reveals to heal and transform you.[168]

What happened when David tuned in, and fixed his thoughts on God? God showed up and opened David's eyes to perceive Truth that transformed his ways of knowing, being, and doing.

Numerous stories describe David's encounters with God on his way *through* scary unknowns, hazardous high-risk situations, and lonely valleys of death. In the secret place of the Almighty,[169] David was supernaturally sustained through the countless unexpected twists and turns life delivered. The Wonderful Counselor[170] provided insight and solutions for seemingly impossible situations. Day after day, year after year, Jehovah Rapha healed David's heart wounds,[171] empowering him to continue fulfilling his purposes in this world.

Do you realize that you are a breath away from your own encounters with the Living God? The greatest desire of your Creator's heart is to enjoy friendship with you. He longs to share conversations together and satisfy the desires of your heart. Like David, He wants to empower you to fully mend, rise up strong, and experience new expressions of His abundant goodness. Father, Son, and Holy Spirit work in tandem, eager to help you listen and hear,[172] to experience Love's fond affection,[173] and to recognize wisdom from above.[174][175]

Do you know that you were created with an innate ability to hear God?[176] God is always speaking and continuously articulate, filling the world with

His speaking voice.[177] When we have trouble hearing, we can simply ask the Holy Spirit to open our ears and help us listen.[178] It's amazing how getting the wax out of our ears, and turning down the noise around us can make it easier to hear God.

I'm deeply grateful for several mentors who inspired me during college and early adulthood to listen for God's voice. Dallas Willard, a brilliant scholar who taught philosophy for nearly fifty years at the University of Southern California, had a profound influence on my spiritual formation. He encouraged me to be open and intentional about developing my listening skills[179] and to practice hearing God. Many years ago, he challenged me in a way that forever changed my way of doing life:

> *Hearing God? A daring idea, some would say--presumptuous and even dangerous. But what if we are made for it? What if the human system simply will not function properly without it? There are good reasons to think it will not. The fine texture as well as the grand movements of life show our need to hear God. Isn't it more presumptuous and dangerous, in fact, to undertake human existence without hearing God?*[180]

Yes, Dr. Willard. I believe it is.

Brother Lawrence, the gentle French monk who wrote *The Practice of the Presence of God* in 1692, spoke of gradually developing the ability to dialogue with God much like we build any other skill worth acquiring. He said, "In order to first form the habit of conversing with God continually, and of referring all that we do to Him, we must first apply ourselves to Him with diligence. After a little such care, we shall find His love inwardly excites us to His presence without difficulty."[181]

C.S. Lewis, a giant among twentieth-century thought leaders, openly acknowledged his personal hunger and challenges to hear God. After years of being steeped in intellectual skepticism, as a teaching fellow in higher academics at Oxford and Cambridge University, Lewis points out the value of starting small and having gentle expectations.

> "When you wake up in the morning all your wishes and hopes for the day rush at you like wild animals. And the first job each morning consists in shoving them all back; in listening to that other voice, taking the other point of view, letting that other, larger, stronger, quieter life come flowing in… We can only do it for moments at first. But from those moments the new sort of life will be spreading through our systems because we are letting Him work in the right place of us."[182]

You and I are designed to flourish in friendship with God. We're invited to think and feel, reason and intuit our way through all the issues of our life *with* God, who knows best how to bring out the finest in us.[183] In ongoing conversation, the Spirit of Truth[184] speaks and acts according to our needs with astounding creativity, always for our highest good in ways that honor God. Truth and peace come in words, pictures, and impressions to the mind fixed on God.[185]

An eternal offer has been extended to you and to me, *"Come now, let us reason together," says the Lord.*[186] In the context of friendly conversation, the Master Mender weaves mysteries and miracles through our stories. C.S. Lewis said this well: "The supernatural is not remote and abstruse. It is a matter of daily and hourly experience, as intimate as breathing. Denial of it depends on a certain absent-mindedness. But this absent-mindedness is in no way surprising."[187]

Many wonderful people are not aware of or accustomed to hearing God in day-to-day life. C.S. Lewis aptly explains the harsh results: "In the conditions produced by a century or so of Naturalism, (a world view which does not acknowledge the supernatural personality of God and miracles) plain men are being forced to bear burdens which plain men were never expected to bear before. We must get the truth for ourselves or go without it.[188]

I wholeheartedly agree. We must acquire the truth for ourselves from the ultimate Source of all Truth and settle for nothing less. As far as I can tell, *now* is the best time to do so, because true growth and education is a kind of never-ending story—a matter of continual beginnings, of habitual fresh starts, of persistent newness.[189]

Do you know that the Holy Spirit revitalizes the contrite heart, turned toward Almighty God? "For this is what the high and exalted One says— he who lives forever, whose name is holy: 'I live in a high and holy place, but also with the one who is contrite and lowly in spirit, to revive the spirit of the lowly and to revive the heart of the contrite.'"[190]

I wonder if you're in a place similar to where I've been before and may find myself again. Are you depleted of hope, feeling like you're barely hanging on by a fragile thread? Are you discouraged or tired of trying to white-knuckle it through the day on dwindling strength? Does it seem like others aren't there for you, or that you're on your own to figure out a way through grief's ruthless overwhelm?

After decades in the counseling office, I'm aware of how frequently men and women silently experience these realities, and I want to reassure you. God is with you right now, in this moment, wanting to empower and sustain you with divine energy.[191] [192]

An Invitation to Action

Would you like to stop a moment and rest awhile in Love's presence? Will you give yourself permission to take a break, breathe, and open your heart to receive whatever you need? I invite you to join me. Let's enter the secret place together.

If you like, take a few deep cleansing breaths to relax and settle in. Fill your lungs fully as you breathe in Love's presence, and then slowly exhale all the tension in your body. Attune your senses to the Spirit of the Living God within and around you and whisper these words with me.

Father of Love, thank you for this safe space with you. Thank you for inviting me to talk with you about what is on my mind. I want to grow in my ability to be open, honest, and willing, to freely share my heart with you and to listen. Help me hear your voice, to sense your nudges, and receive your goodness. I silence every other voice from disrupting our time together. Let Your voice be the loudest one I hear.

I need help to keep going. I can't do this alone. Please infuse my being with supernatural grace. Fill me afresh with Your Holy Spirit.[193] Energize the cells of my body, the feelings of my heart, the faculties of my mind, and the determination of my will with your life-giving power. Permeate my weakness with strength from heaven. Resurrect the withered lifeless areas in me, the ones that I can't even identify or find words to describe. I'm open to receive your peace, comfort, and every good gift You have for me.[194]

Thank you for inviting me to draw near, and for tenderly wrapping me in healing Love. Help me learn to relax and feel at home in your presence.[195] I trust You to teach me how to talk with you in ways that renew my mind and mend my heart. Guide and sustain me, while we walk through this dark valley together into new beginnings. And Lord... (Feel free to add anything else on your heart.)

There's no need to rush anywhere right now. Linger awhile in the peaceful place of Love's embrace. Notice how calm and safe your body can feel in quiet stillness with God. Pay attention to what you sense and try to memorize it. Then take a moment to jot down a few highlights from your time with God.

When you're ready, we'll move forward and explore *Love Talks* —a gentle, grace-filled space where you'll learn how to release your grief and open your heart to receive from God in practical, healing ways. As we walk through this model together, once again, you'll see how deep heartache can be touched by redeeming love and radically transformed.

> *How I wish, wish, wish, that a dozen or more persons who are trying to hold God endlessly in mind, would all write their experiences so that each would know what the other was finding as a result! The results I think would astound the world.*[196]

My husband passed away after a brief, fierce fight with cancer. Before he got sick, we planned to move to another state. Not long after he passed, I sensed God nudging me to make the big move. But our son and daughter were teens. Leaving their friends and the only home they'd ever known within a year of losing their dad, didn't seem like a wise choice. Yet, I kept hearing God say, "It's the right move, and right time."

During the kids' spring break, we travel across state lines, looked at property and visited a church. My teenagers were non-committal, voicing pros and cons about moving to a rural area, vastly different from our current suburban life.

I worked up the courage to tell my 15-year-old son that I believed God wanted us to move. He completely lost it, sobbing long and hard about more losses. My heart broke all over again. Sitting on the floor with him, I held him close, and we cried together.

Through streaming tears, I silently told God how much I wanted to do what I sensed he wanted me to do. I surrendered the plans and timing again, willing to put the move on hold if it would harm or hinder my children's healing. I desperately needed wisdom.

As I poured out my heart, I sensed a clear impression: "Daughter, I love your son more than you can imagine. Trust me. I am speaking to him, too. I will guide and comfort him. Press forward with your plans. Trust me."

So, I did. We continued to plan, talk openly and pray together about our hopes and fears. God did what he said he would do. While we were wrapping up the school year, God reassured my son in many ways. Before we left the state, he told me he felt secure and at peace that life would be okay where we were headed.

That was over a year ago. My son is adjusting well, healing from his father's death, thriving with friends, and loving life. Older men in our community have befriended him like dad figures. My daughter is flourishing, enjoying a full ride scholarship to a private school. We continue to be overwhelmed by God's amazing goodness. I'm thankful that I listened to God and acted. If I hadn't, we would have missed out on so many amazing blessings!

O our God, we do not know what to do but we are looking to you for help.
2 Chronicles 20:12, NLT

LOVE TALK *Rachelle Rodriguez*

15

RELEASE AND RECEIVE

God's voice says to you, "I want to see you come closer to me and experience the joy and peace of My presence. I want to give you a new heart and a new spirit. All that is mine is yours. Just trust me and let me be your God."

Henry Nouwen

One of the most painful parts of grief is, perhaps, the tangled web of great sadness, lonely longings, and persistent fatigue. Grief, like a dark fog, overtakes your faculties and becomes what you tend to see and feel most. Anguish is determined to run the show, like a selfish child demanding his own way. Not only are you consumed with sorrow over what is missing, but you're preoccupied with misery's shadow or reflection, the fact that you don't merely suffer, but have to keep on thinking about the fact that you suffer.[197]

In this weakened vulnerable state, it's difficult to see and think clearly. We're more susceptible to harmful influences that, at other times, we can typically recognize and deflect. I discovered my own vulnerability firsthand, multiple times after Nathan's traumatic accident. The first blindside happened on his third day in the Pediatric Intensive Care Unit.

Stories about Nathan aired across local and national news media—for ten days.

Talk radio stations opened their phone lines, inviting public opinions, and the floodgates of judgment burst wide open. Critics wasted no time. Their words flew fast and cruel, cutting deep.

Angry voices, hostile to the sacredness of life, rushed to condemn us. They accused us of everything imaginable: willful neglect, abandonment, and parental failure. We were stunned and humiliated. Reeling in the vulnerable haze of our heartbreak, the fiery serpent bit.

Never in my life did I imagine we'd be fighting this kind of battle—not only for Nathan's life, but for our sense of integrity. Shame and blame slithered in from every angle, whispering lies in the dark: *Good parents wouldn't let this happen! If God really loved you, He would have prevented this…*

And yet, into that violent despair, God blew a tiny spark.

The hospital room was heavy with trauma. I sat beside Nathan, gently holding his hand, my eyes closed and head resting on the back of the chair. Bone-deep exhaustion had settled in. I couldn't recall ever feeling so utterly emptied and undone.

That's when I sensed someone in the room. I opened my eyes, and there she was: the hospital social worker assigned to Nathan's case. She was petite, maybe five-feet tall with shoes on—but there in the doorway, she stood strong with the quiet force of a lighthouse in a wicked storm. There was nothing timid about her. She radiated energy from within with a resolve that cut through my gloom like a laser.

"I had to come tell you to stay off all media," she said firmly. "Don't listen to a word they're saying. They don't know what they're talking about!"

In that moment, her fierce compassion collided with my despair and cracked it open. It was as if a window had been thrown wide that allowed the winds of the Spirit to sweep in, blow away the lies and revive me.

That's the power of someone who's willing to stand in the storm with you—not to fix, but to see, to protect, and to believe when you've forgotten how. Mary's voice that day didn't just defend us. It pulled me out of a cesspool of shame and reminded me that truth still lives, and love still wins.

Here's the point I want to make: when we're willing to be with someone in their pain, we begin to understand the immense, transforming power of simply being present. The darkness is real. But so is our light.

Can you see it? How the messiest, meanest moments in life expose just how much we need each other—how desperately we need to be seen, heard, and held? There are no do-it-yourself kits for a broken heart. Healing doesn't happen solo. Healing is relational.

And sometimes, all it takes to begin afresh is one person brave enough to show up.

* * *

Breaking Lies and Owning Truth

"Ask God to show you one lie that you believe about yourself and write it down." That's how the leader opened the training session.

An unanticipated answer instantly came to mind: *You're too old.*

Huh! The thought caught me by complete surprise, and yet, somehow, I knew it rang true.

"Now, ask God when that lie took root," the leader said.

Something strange happened on the heels of that invitation. I spontaneously recalled a business mastermind group I had participated in years before. The memory was clear. I was sitting at a circular table in a hotel, surrounded by successful entrepreneurs from various countries around the world. You'd likely recognize the names of a few of the higher-level influencers.

A handsome, charismatic young man, whom I'll call Nick, talked about the explosive growth he was experiencing in his educational courses. In one year, he moved from training five or six people in a six-week program to several hundred at a time. Business was booming and transformation was happening all around him. That got my attention!

Curious to hear more, I approached Nick during a break and asked him about his work. He lit up, eager to share, and explained that he had created a multi-layered series of educational trainings. When I asked who typically attended his courses, he replied, "Mostly people who are down-and-out—vulnerable individuals who've been wounded by people and hardship." Then he launched into an elevator pitch: *"I help hurting people learn occult practices that bring power and relief."*

His words hit hard. They were confident, polished, and deeply troubling. What Nick offered sounded like hope, but it was rooted in something far darker. Vulnerable people were being lured into a shadow realm – one not designed to heal, but to siphon away whatever vestiges of life remained in their injured souls.[198]

Later that afternoon, I recall looking around the room and noticing that 90 percent of the participants shared something in common. They were a decade or more behind me in age. Only a few individuals were older. I don't recall drawing any specific conclusions, but I believe God was showing me that the lie 'I'm too old' took root then and there.

Now, turn your focus toward God," the leader said. "Imagine yourself handing your paper—the one with the lie you identified—to Jesus. Watch what He does with it, and write down what you see."

So, I did and made a few notes: Jesus playfully tossed the paper over his shoulder and burst out laughing. I'm not talking about a quiet little chuckle. I'm talking big, carbonated laughter that keeps rolling up and over like a fountain. At that moment, warmth rushed through me. Jesus grinned and said, "Watch Me!"

I'm not exactly sure of everything that shifted in that brief moment, but one thing became clear: after a lifetime in a culture that idolizes youth, the lie, "I'm too old," lost its hold on me. Something broke free inside. I felt a fresh sense of freedom being comfortable in my own skin, and embracing this season of life as a bona fide senior. Seeing Jesus laugh from deep in His belly over that *age* hangup did my heart good!

I want to pause here and invite you to notice something.

In just a brief moment with God, I let go of a lie I hadn't even realized was holding me back. God gently brought it to the surface, and with it, the grace to trade it for something true. In that sacred exchange, I saw an image of Jesus laughing—*really* laughing—from deep in His belly, over something that, to Him, was completely absurd and irrelevant. That moment of clarity was unlike anything I'd ever experienced. It felt like a holy breath of fresh air. Even now, it still makes me smile.

It was a glimpse into what's possible when we come before God with an honest, open, willing heart—ready to release what weighs us down and receive perspective He longs to give. It's a picture of prayer—not just words, but an honest, vulnerable exchange that changes us.

Tish Harrison Warren captures it beautifully when she says that prayer is the willingness to enter into ambiguity and vulnerability—but not just any ambiguity. It's the vulnerability of discovering we are deeply loved, and learning, again and again, how to receive that love and trust it to be true.[199]

So, we lift our hearts to heaven once more: Dear Lord, we need Your help. Would you increase our capacity to release and receive? Teach us to trust Your creative grace to meet us in every moment, and to set us free, again and again.

An Invitation to Action

- Ask God to bring to mind one lie that you currently believe about yourself. Write down the first idea that comes to mind in your prayer notebook.

- Invite God to show you when you began believing the lie. Think back through the timeline of your life with open curiosity. If it's important for you to know, the truth will come. Your *knower* will know. If not, no worries. It's the Holy Spirit's job to reveal. It's your job to ask and receive.

- In your mind's eye see yourself handing the lie you wrote in your notebook over to Jesus. What does He do with it? Ask what this means, listen, and take notes.

- Ask God for wisdom. What truth cancels that lie? Write down your insights.

- Ask God if there is anything else He wants to bring to your attention. Don't censor or second guess what may seem unknown or different. Sometimes God uses the unfamiliar or an element of surprise to get your attention and highlight that you didn't come up with that idea on your own. Let me offer two personal examples that illustrate what I mean.

Midway through my husband's career, he weathered a major management transition at work. Given the turn of events, we wondered if God might lead us to move elsewhere.

One morning while talking with God about the uncertainties ahead, the following words came to mind, "John is ballast."

"Ballast?" I wondered. "What is ballast?" I wasn't familiar with the term.

As a little girl, I used to ask my mom and dad the meaning of words. Can you guess their standard reply?

"Look it up in the dictionary, and tell us what you find."

Having learned that lesson well, I pulled Merriam-Webster off the shelf and discovered that ballast is the heavy material placed low in a vessel to improve steadiness and stability.

One little whisper quieted my concerns about future unknowns. I figured for the time being, we were staying put. And that's how the story happened to play out.

LOVE TALK

I completed writing book three, in a five-book series. Eager to begin the next project, I wrote down three ideas and asked God for wisdom on which topic to pursue: "Do we go with idea #1, #2, or #3?"

The only thing that came to mind was, "STOP."

I paused and blinked. Stop? That felt strange. The contract was signed. The timeline was set. I'm a woman who keeps her word and I don't back out of commitments. I figured I must've been distracted, so I quieted my mind, silenced every other voice, and asked again, this time more focused: "Okay Lord, what do You think—idea #1, #2, or #3?"

Once more, the answer came: "STOP."

It made no sense. There were financial obligations, deadlines, and people depending on me. Still puzzled, I decided to bring it up with my husband, John, later that evening. He's as steady and committed as they come, and I assumed he'd echo my sense of duty to follow through.

But as we stood side by side at the sink, washing dishes, I told him about my conversation with God and how confused I felt. Without even hesitating, he said, "You better go with what you hear God saying."

That's when I knew—I had to make the call.

With sweaty palms, I phoned the senior editor the next day. I explained what I'd sensed in prayer. He wasn't thrilled and asked to meet in person the following week. By the time we finished talking, he accepted the reality and asked me to let him know when I was ready to write again. I walked away feeling sad to disappoint the team—but peacefully relieved, knowing I had responded well to God.

And then, six weeks later, an 18-wheeler barreled down a hill and slammed into our daughter in stop-and-go freeway traffic. The year that followed was filled with agony, uncertainty, and emotional weight I could never have predicted. Looking back, I can't imagine carrying the pressure of a writing contract during that season. God, in His mercy, had prepared the road ahead before the adversities ever came.

But that's not all Two years later, out of the blue, the publishing team decided on their own to repackage the first three books of that series into a brand-new release —**The Power of Letting Go.** *Only God!*

LOVE TALK

An Invitation to Action

One of my favorite routines is finding a quiet space where I can fully relax and let go of the day's tension from head to toe. Once I'm still and calm, I imagine God drawing near, wrapping me in a soft comforting blanket of peace. I picture us alone together in a beautiful place—maybe sitting together in an alpine meadow filled with wildflowers, or a sandy beach near warm, blue water.

In that sacred place, I imagine the Father, Son, and Holy Spirit forming a circle of love around me—moving in sync, creating perfect harmony in the atmosphere, and filling my awareness with all that is good.

Here God and I talk together. I ask questions, I listen, and I write down what comes to mind. I'd love for you to try this simple practice, too. I invite you to experiment with a Love Talk, keeping these simple guidelines in mind:

- Find a quiet place to calm your heart-soul-mind-body with purposeful breathing.

- Humbly surrender yourself and all of your concerns to God.

- Silence any thoughts not in full agreement with the Spirit of the Living God and Truth.

- Pick one issue that is on your mind and freely write your thoughts and feelings, expressing whatever is inside without evaluation or judgment.

- Ask God a question, take time to listen, and write down what comes to mind.[200][201]

- Ask God for three confirmations about what you sense God saying to you (through Scripture, wise friends, circumstances, inner peace, Holy Spirit intuitions, etc.)

The secret place of God's love chamber yields hidden treasure.[202] There is nothing arbitrary about what the Holy Spirit illumines or random about the grace gifts he shares with you.[203] Precision and strategy are woven through what God says, when and how He says it, and the ways He exchanges our ashes for beauty, and mourning for blessing.[204] God's supreme goodness is found in the details.

I recently stumbled upon an entry in an old prayer notebook from years ago. Apparently, I was exhausted and discouraged at the time. Hoping for a lift out of my flat funk, I began my prayer with a genuine question. What I sensed God say is written in italics.

God, I'm weary, worn out from all the pressing needs around me.

Could you remind me of something you love about me?

The way you honor me pursuing excellence.

Wow... I did not see that coming. Thank you for noticing my effort. Sometimes I wonder if it even matters. Is there anything else you want me to know?

You're tired and don't feel well. Rest in a slower rhythm. Faster is not better. We'll finish on time.

Oh... I see. Thank you for reminding me to set a gentler pace, to tame my tempo. I feel peace now. I can rest in Your timing, Father. Would you breathe fresh wind into my soul? Lift me beyond my own natural inclinations and help me to love You, and others, and myself as You do. Open my eyes to see the beauty that You see. I don't want to miss a single thing. I love you so much!

> *May the Lord lead your hearts into a full understanding and expression of the love of God and the patient endurance that comes from Christ.*
> 2 Thes. 3:5, NLT.

LOVE TALK

It was no accident that I stumbled onto that old journal entry. I definitely needed a kind nudge to reset my pace and remember that God did exactly what he said he would do in that season. We successfully hit a challenging deadline together, right on time.

Friend, let this sink in: the magnitude of God's grace isn't based on your performance or mine. It's not about how good we've been, how much we've done, or how worthy we feel. It's not about us at all. It's about Him—our Creator—whose love is beyond measure, whose affection for us is unshakable.

You were created in love, by Love Himself. God's love hasn't faded and never will. The promise still stands—unchanged by time or circumstance:

> *The one who obeys (hears and responds)*[205] *me is the one who loves me; and because he loves me, my Father will love him; and I will too, and I will reveal myself to him.*[206]

Please don't miss this beautiful promise. God wants to be known by you. He's not distant or disinterested—He's near, and His heart is open wide. He longs to show you more of who He is… more of who you truly are… and the healing friendship that's always been waiting for you.

No matter where you've been or what you're carrying, just turn to God. One step toward Him is enough—ask Him to show you He's real, and with the eyes of your heart, you'll see: He's already coming toward you with compassion, ready to lead you into a life of freedom, fullness, and love beyond anything you've known.

I was not a happy camper!

We spent the day building our sleep shelters out of forest debris that we collected from the area. My body and mind were depleted, running on fumes . Extreme exhaustion set in after living 2 months in the wilderness for specialized training. (For context - I'm not an outdoorsy person, and I like comfort.)

Simply executing the day's routine felt like slogging through quicksand. Working on my shelter with such limited capacity was daunting. I kept telling myself, "This is fun! You can do this, Michelle! You've got this!"

It didn't help. I just wanted to leave.

Then came a whisper, *The greater the battle the greater the breakthrough.*

That kept me going for awhile, but a few hours later I was silently throwing a hissy fit as I squeezed into a tight, cold, dark shelter to try to sleep for the night. The ground was hard. I was exposed to dangers that only God knew lurked near. Comfort was nowhere to be found. The training had whittlled me down to my most raw parts.

In my misery I asked God, "What do you want me to know?

Being uncomfortable isn't an emergency, came the reply.

God's answer hit the bulls eye and empowered me to level up. I carry this liberating truth wherever I go and continue to use it to this day.

LOVE TALK

Michelle D.

16

GRACE GIFTS

Your primary contact with God is through your mind, and what you do with your mind is the most important choice you have to make.[207]

Dallas Willard

I want to introduce you to someone who discovered *Love Talks* in the middle of deep heartbreak.

When she first heard about the idea of having a two-way conversation with God, she was pretty skeptical. Honestly, it felt foreign and a little uncomfortable. But she was open to trying it—just once. And something incredible happened: God tenderly met her right in her pain and poured out so much goodness.[208]

Much to her surprise, love started to drive out a fear she'd carried since she was a little girl.[209]

Sandy is a middle-aged woman who's struggled with sadness and anxiety for as long as she can remember. She reached out to me after losing Cooper, her beloved dog of 19 years. He had been her constant companion and comfort through the years, the one who greeted her at the door when no one else did. Cooper didn't just fill a space in her home; he filled a space in her heart that others couldn't reach. Without him, the house felt painfully empty.

But it wasn't just Cooper's absence. Sandy's adult daughter—who had been struggling with her mental health—cut off all contact. No explanation. No discussion. Just silence. And that silence left Sandy feeling helpless, anxious, and riddled with guilt. Was it something she said? Something she didn't say? Her mind couldn't stop spinning, running over every moment, every word, trying to make sense of the disconnection. The weight of not knowing was unbearable.

For Sandy, the grief came in layers—sharp, overlapping waves that made it hard to breathe. Her feelings about Cooper were tangled-up with a fear that her daughter might never come back. The burden was way too much for anyone to bear alone.

That's when Sandy reached out—exhausted, and longing for some kind of hope.

Over a handful of video calls, I gently walked with Sandy through some simple but powerful truths—about grief, emotional healing, and what real transformation can look like.

One thing I kept coming back to is this: healing happens best when we do it together with *Triune Love*—Father, Son, and Holy Spirit. Why? Because God's nature is pure love. His grace, His creativity, His presence—it all works together to bring us into a place of abundant wholeness.[210]

God isn't far away. He's right here. He's ready to help you see what needs healing, and to give you exactly what you need to take the next step.

That next step often looks like surrender and trust. And if I'm being honest—trust is where things can get hard. It's the very place where resistance tends to show up every which way. The darkness rivals for the souls of men and women and doesn't give up easily.[211][212]

But trusting faith digs in, holds on, clings tight, and says, "I don't care what happens, I'm holding on to God!"[213] And that's where Love begins to do its deepest work.

Allow me to share a bit of Sandy's story. Sandy grew up as an only child in a home that felt emotionally cold and unpredictable. Her mother, though physically present, was often self-absorbed and rarely gave Sandy the kind of warm, affirming attention every child needs. Instead, she focused heavily on rules and was quick to point out Sandy's mistakes, leaving her feeling like she could never quite measure up.

Her father struggled with alcoholism. He was around, but emotionally distant—unable to offer the comfort or connection Sandy longed for.

The one bright spot early in her life was her grandmother. Sandy adored her because she was warm, nurturing, and consistent—the one person who made her feel truly seen and safe.

These three individuals—her critical mother, absent father, and loving grandmother—shaped the emotional landscape of Sandy's childhood.

It's important to remember that our need for emotional healing often goes deeper than our most recent grief or loss. While current heartbreak, such as the death of a loved one or the pain of a rejection is deeply real, it's rarely the whole story.

More often than not, today's pain is intertwined with older, unresolved wounds—experiences from childhood or previously where our emotional needs weren't met. These earlier hurts can quietly shape the way we experience our present-day losses.

That was true for Sandy. While she was grieving the loss of Cooper and the painful silence from her daughter, she was also feeling the ache of earlier losses—growing up in an environment where love, affirmation, and nurturing were scarce. That kind of emotional deprivation leaves marks in the soul.

When I talk about "injuries," I'm referring to those moments during childhood when we felt invisible, unimportant, dismissed, or mistreated. Times when, from a child's limited perspective, we formed beliefs about ourselves, about God, and about others that weren't true but felt real. We may have made conclusions such as, *"I'm not worthy,"* or *"Love always leaves,"* or *"I'm on my own."*

These wounds don't just disappear over time. The body holds on to them. They live in our nervous systems, and show up in our reactions in our relationships. And to cope, we often develop protective walls—defenses that may have helped us survive our past, but now keep us from fully healing and connecting.

Recognizing this isn't about blaming the past—it's about compassion. It's about understanding why we hurt the way we do, and gently inviting God into those hidden places so we can finally begin to heal.

During one of our conversations, Sandy opened up about how the last couple of weeks had been especially hard.

She said, *"I've been hit with this awful anxiety that seems to come out of nowhere. It doesn't make any sense. I'm an educated, professional woman—but the moment I start thinking about trying something new, or aiming for a bigger goal, this wave of anxiety shows up. It's like my body intuitively knows something bad will happen if I move forward. I get a "strong gut knowing" that*

I'll fail, or things will fall apart. No matter how much I try to talk myself out of it, the fear doesn't budge."

"What do you do when that happens?" I asked.

"Oh, that's easy!" she replied. "I *stop trying* so that something bad won't happen."

"Where did that come from?" I wondered aloud.

A blank stare washed over Sandy's face followed by long moments of deep thought. Breaking the silence, she shrugged her shoulders, threw up her hands, and exclaimed, "I don't have a clue!"

"Well, it's completely okay that you don't have a clue," I responded. "If knowing where the anxiety comes from is necessary for your healing, God will show you what you need to know at the right time. He's kind and gentle that way."

Sandy leaned back, sank down into her chair, sighed, and said, "I guess, but it's just so frustrating!"

I understood Sandy's bewilderment, having experienced it myself and witnessed it in many others through the years. Her struggle was beyond the common flat blah and low motivation that naturally accompanies grief fatigue. She truly wanted to move forward, but fear had the upper hand in driving her decisions.

Why did that supercharged anxiety seemingly burst out of nowhere, unannounced, and larger than life? Why was she floundering, unable to set objectives that her family and friends were convinced she was capable of achieving? I wondered if experiences from childhood, feelings she *caught* from others and internalized, held her hostage.

To her credit, Sandy refused to keep putting-up with the troublesome anxiety and brought it out into the light. She wanted to practice something she learned:

What we reveal can be healed.

I reassured Sandy, telling her, what I now pass on to you: God cares deeply about the deprivations and heartaches you've suffered through life. He aches with compassion over any wounds and losses you've endured. Father, Son, and Holy Spirit are touched by the *feelings* of your weaknesses[214] (notice that word feelings), including all the emotions stored in the mental maps beyond conscious awareness, held in the cells of your body.

Rest assured, the Holy Spirit knows best how to help you in your weakness.[215] With extraordinary creativity and greater precision than the world's most renowned heart surgeon, the Lover of your soul longs for an invitation to partner with you in repairing and regenerating your emotions with healing grace.

Even when you don't know what to say or how to pray, the Holy Spirit is talking with Triune Love about what you need. There is not the slightest confusion in God's mind about all you've experienced, and He is never at a loss about how to communicate on your behalf.[216]

"Sandy, I'm wondering if we could try something together. Are you open to inviting God into this conversation, to help you take the next step toward freedom?"

"I don't know. What does that look like?" she asked apprehensively.

I offered a simple explanation: "Have you ever done a three-way call with co-workers or friends? (Sandy had done so many times. It was easy for her to connect with the metaphor). It's a bit like doing a three-way phone call. You and I are talking together, and what I'd like to do is invite God to join our conversation, to help us explore what's going on inside.[217] We'll ask

God for perspective and wisdom about the hidden fear that keeps popping up and shutting down your growth. God knows better than anyone how the complex connections in your heart-soul-mind-body work together. He has a way of cutting through layers of confusion with grace and truth[218] like nobody else. Healing your grief is best orchestrated by God.[219] We can all work together. Is that OK with you?"

Sandy said she was willing to try, as I led the way into a conversation with God. The following sequence of events unfolded.

Sandy and I took a few deep breaths together to relax in the moment, and I prayed:

> *Lord, thank you for Sandy and her longing to grow and become everything you created her to be. Father, Son, and Holy Spirit, we invite You to join our conversation. Thank You for being here with us. You're always with us. Before we even ask, You know that we want your help and need your wisdom.[220]*
>
> *We come to you now, fixing our eyes on you.[221] Open our ears to hear and our eyes to see what You want us to know. We silence every voice other than the Spirit of the Living God from influencing our conversation.[222] In our imagination, we envision You here in this room with us, and acknowledge the deep compassion you feel for Sandy's heartache. I ask You to lead us into grace and truth as we talk things over with You.[223]*

I explained the next step to Sandy,

> *By faith, we're going to believe that God will speak to us. I'll start by asking God a question, and then I'd like you to describe any words, pictures, insights, or Holy Spirit-led intuitions that come to your awareness. There's no need to analyze, overthink, or critique what comes to mind. Simply allow the process to unfold and verbalize what you sense. You're safe in Love's presence.[224]*

Sandy nodded in understanding and agreement.

> *Lord, we ask You for wisdom.*[225] *What do you want Sandy to understand about the anxiety she was overwhelmed by this week?*

Sandy responded, "What comes to mind is a trip to my grandparents' home. I recall riding on a train with my mother to see my grandmother and grandfather in South Dakota. I was a toddler and liked to hold onto the edge of the coffee table in front of their couch and scoot around it.

Grandma decorated the middle of the table with pretty collectibles. One afternoon, I reached out to touch one, and my mother slapped my hand. I reached again and Mama slapped my hand even harder. Grandma stood back telling Mama, 'Let her have them, dear. She can't hurt anything. If they break, they break. I'm not attached to them.'

Mama said, 'No! Sandy has to learn that she can't touch certain things!'

Each time I reached, Mama slapped. This went back and forth until I finally plopped down on the floor crying hysterically. Mama used to tell the story at family gatherings about how she 'taught me a lesson.' She said I was so persistent she slapped my hands 'until they were beet red.' As usual, Grandma always chimed in with her perspective, 'I think you were too hard on her, darling.'

Grandma was my loving soft place to land."

Ahhh, so your grandma was a safe person?

"Yes! Grandma was the only safe person during my early years."

Do you recall experiencing any feelings when your mother slapped your hands?

"I sense a vague sting right now, a tingling on the top of my hands. It's like it's right on the edge."

Sandy paused a few seconds, self-consciously laughed, and said, "I'm thinking this is really silly; like I'm making it all up, and the stinging can't actually be real."

(Notice how Sandy shifted from feeling memories into analysis, moving from emotion to reason. Intellectualizing is a common defense mechanism we use to avoid feeling emotional pain. I responded by simply reassuring her.)

Sandy, you're safe. You asked God to speak to you and to guide you into truth. There's no need to second guess what you sense. (In the moments that followed, a dense fog seemed to lift for the first time in years. Sandy began to see with her spiritual eyes and was able to connect her thoughts with her feelings.)

"My hands hurt, and I feel sad. But I don't know why I feel sad. I'm confused. Did I do something wrong? What did I do wrong?"

(The mind perceives more clearly in a peaceful state. When Sandy's feelings intensified, we shifted momentarily so as to breathe and quiet the heart-soul-mind-body.)

Sandy, we're going to pause and settle back into a place of peace. Take a few deep cleansing breaths and allow your body to calm. Shift your attention back to God. He knows all there is to know about the situation. You have His full love and attention right now. Are you able to envision God here with you?

"Yes."

What do you notice?

"Jesus is sitting next to me."

Do you sense anything specific?

"I feel joy coming from Him, like he's glad to be here and wants to stay."

OK. Sandy, picture yourself placing all the sadness and confusion from the incident at your grandma's house into a physical object that you can hold in your hands. It can be any item you choose that symbolizes your grief. Are you able to envision a tangible item?

"Yes."

Can you describe it for me?

"It looks like a ball made of papier-mâché, wrapped in a lot of layered strips. The strips are light tan, similar to the color of masking tape. The papier-mâché ball is huge compared to me. I can barely wrap both of my arms around it. It's probably the size of a volleyball in real life, but I'm little and the ball is enormous in my small hands."

What does it feel like?

"It actually feels kind of rough, scratchy, and prickly on my hands."

How heavy is it?

"It's not particularly heavy. It's just bulky and awkward to hold."

Can you picture yourself handing the ball to Jesus sitting beside you?

"Yes."

What does Jesus do when you hand it over?

"Jesus looks at the ball. Now he's smiling at me and tucking it under one arm."

What does that mean?

"It's not my burden to carry anymore. He's got it. Now he's throwing the ball onto a big pile of garbage. (Sandy laughs.) Oh, that's funny. My first thought is, 'Oh, Jesus don't throw it away.' Now WHY would I think THAT?!"

That's a great question. Why don't you ask Him?

Sandy thought silently.

"Hmmm... I think it's because it's been a part of me for so long, that it sort of feels like He's throwing me away."

Do you want to ask Him if that's the truth?

"He's letting me know it's not true. He'll never throw me away. I'm his precious child. He wants me to feel free from carrying the burden. He knows it's big and sticky, and difficult for me to let it go. He's reassuring me that I don't have to do it myself."

Would you like to ask for help?

"Yes! Jesus, will you help me live without this burden? I can sense He's here to help me. He wants me to trust Him. He knows my struggles and He doesn't seem disappointed in me. He's not critical, scolding or lecturing me. He's reassuring me that I can trust Him and that He will keep helping me trust Him."

(I recognized this was a pivotal moment because trust was especially challenging for Sandy due to childhood trauma. We lingered momentarily until the Holy Spirit prompted another question.)

Sandy, how do you want to respond to Jesus?

She paused a few moments and replied anxiously, "I'm not sure. There's nothing there. Nothing is there... NOTHING. I'm blocked. I'm stuck."

(The perception of "nothing there" was accurate. The interpretation of "being blocked" was not. As we continued, the Holy Spirit guided Sandy into truth.)

Sandy, the truth is you are not blocked. You're in motion. You're in the middle of a conversation with God. At the very core of that big ball covered in layers of sticky stuff is the dread of something bad happening. You handed that burden over to Jesus. He took it, tucked it under his arm, and then threw it on a garbage pile. Has anything bad happened?

(In the following moments God began to redefine Sandy's reality in new pictures on the screen of her mind.)

"No…" she replied. "Wait! Wait a minute! What is that? Jesus, what am I seeing? It's a hole, an empty space. The place where the burden used to be is bare. There's nothing there now!"

Yes! Sandy, why don't you ask God to fill the empty space with his love? In your own words tell God that you're willing to receive everything He knows you need to heal. Be open to receiving whatever gift God may have for you.

"Jesus, is there something You want to offer to replace my burden?"

(Following a long pause, Sandy began to describe what she experienced.)

"Wow! Jesus is peeling away the layered strips covering the ball. One by one, around, and around, He's unwrapping the sticky coverings all the way down to the core. He takes something from inside the ball, and hands me a small figurine. It's one of the pretty porcelains that were on my grandma's coffee table! Oh! Wow! I feel warmth spreading through my chest. I can see my grandmother smiling! Wow! Jesus let me see my grandmother smiling!" (Sandy sat silently, in awe of God's goodness.)[226]

Linger there a while and soak in God's presence, Sandy. Let God's love permeate and imprint every part of your being. (After several minutes passed, I asked if there was more.)

Sandy, does anything else come to your awareness?

"Yes. I see the little girl crying, but she's not crying in pain. She's crying because she's overcome with joy and relief!"

Lovely! Go ahead and ask God what that means.

"He's reassuring me again. He wants me to know that whatever I've lost, He will restore. No matter how small and insignificant it may seem, or how huge or awful it may be, Jesus loves me so much, he will do that for me.

There's something else. I see that the figurine is very small compared to that big awkward ball. It's light, easy to hold, and fits my hand just right."[227]

That's beautiful, Sandy. God is the kindest person you will ever meet! By any chance do you have an object at home that can serve as a symbolic reminder of this conversation with God? Something tangible you can display and easily notice throughout the day?

"Yes! I have the perfect reminder! (She left to retrieve something from another room and then held it up for me to see.) When Cooper died, a dear friend gave me this small wooden figurine of an angel cradling a little dog close to her heart.

It was such a simple gift, but it deeply touched me. Now, when I look at it, I'll remember how much I loved Cooper—and how much God loves me.

It will help me hold on to the memory of what it felt like to give my grief to Jesus… to see my grandmother's warm smile… and to feel Jesus's joy over being with me."

That's fabulous! When you notice the figurine, pause and become aware of Love warmly embracing you just as you are, in that moment. Thank God for being mighty in you[228] *and for helping you become ever more sensitive and responsive to His presence.*[229] *Thank Him for orchestrating your healing. Tell him aloud so that your ears hear it, too: "I trust You, I trust You, I trust You, to complete the good work You are doing in me."*[230][231]

"OK! I will do that! Oh, I noticed something else that's really different—I feel a unique kind of joy that I've never experienced before. It's like Jesus is happy because I'm happy!"

Sandy and I laughed out loud, and I said, "Yes, ma'am! Never doubt it for a second, because that's the truth!"[232]

Sandy was on her way forward, in a new rhythmic dance with the master Mender. She continued to practice opening her heart to Love, releasing her burdens, and receiving God's grace. The process was deliberate, routine, gentle, and relaxed.

Over the following weeks, God marvelously showed up again and again. The evidence continues to fill the pages of Sandy's prayer notebooks. You'll find another of Sandy's Love Talks at the end of this chapter.

Months later, Sandy stood in her kitchen talking to Jesus about something that was troubling her. As she prayed, an image came to mind: she saw herself playfully bouncing the papier-mâché ball across the kitchen floor to Jesus. In that moment, a deep sense of love and calm washed over her. That experience spoke powerfully to me—it revealed the compassion of the Great Physician,[233] who heals the brokenhearted and rewires the nervous system while redeeming painful memories. Little by little, stitch by stitch, Sandy was on the mend.

Do you feel a gentle stirring in your heart?

Maybe a quiet longing to truly *experience* God—not just know about Him, but to develop a friendship and let Him carefully guide you through your grief to newness of life?

If so, don't ignore that longing. It's an invitation. Why not call out to Him?[234] He's listening, and He will answer.[235] He longs to share with you beautiful, hidden things you haven't yet known.[236]

And please, don't overcomplicate this. It's simpler than we often think. Just speak to Him—honestly, from where you are—and then pause to listen. The answers may not come all at once, but they *will* come.

Even if this kind of conversation with God is new to you—or feels uncertain—there is no step you can take toward God that Love won't meet with grace and goodness.

An Invitation to Action

1. For the next seven days, take a five-minute break during the day to practice silence. Set a timer and focus on breathing deeply (B.O.P.) until you reach a peaceful state. Then, ask God to give you one word or phrase that will bring comfort to your grieving heart. Write down the specific answers you receive each day.

2. After you've gathered your list of words or phrases, ask God if there's anything more He wants you to understand about them. Is there a specific action step He's leading you to take? Spend some quiet time listening, and write down your insights in your prayer journal.

3. Take one small step toward what you sense God inviting you into.[237]

I think God sometimes uses the completely inexplicable events in our lives to point us toward Him. We get to decide each time whether we will lean in toward what is unfolding and say yes or back away. The folks who were following Jesus in Galilee got to decide the same thing each day because there was no road map, no program, and no certainty. All they had was this person, an idea, and an invitation to come and see.

Bob Goff

Jesus met me this morning beside the pool at Coral Baja. I was nestled in my favorite lounge chair on the north side, under the shade of a cabana umbrella. At first, I thought it was Bob sitting beside me. But when I looked again, it wasn't Bob at all—it was Jesus. He wore swim trunks and looked completely at ease.

I was surprised to see Him in the shade and asked why He wasn't out in the sun. He smiled and said, "I don't have a need for the sun. I am the Son." We both laughed the kind of chuckles that feel light in your chest.

"Sandy, look around—what do you see?," he asked.

I scanned the area around us. "I see the ocean, the surf, the sand, waves crashing, and beach cabanas. And—wait—Mama Mia's Café… What? Mama Mia's? Hold on! – I see my mom! Here? Now?!"

My breath caught in my throat. Anxiety swelled. "My mother?!—Really?!—Jesus, I'm not ready for this!"

Jesus didn't move. He lounged peacefully beside me, eyes closed, and gently said, "Take your time, Sandy. . .I'm here with you."

Mom slowly walked toward us. Instinctively I began to rise, but Jesus reached out and said, "Wait. Sandy, let her come to you."

Mom sat beside me vibrant and youthful—looking to be in her twenties, dressed in simple, elegant clothes from the 1940s. Her beauty was natural and effortless. I smiled and said, "You still have your Betty Grable legs." She laughed aloud, full of life.

On the outside, I wore a smile. But inside, my walls were up—as always. I didn't know how to act, uncertain about how to receive this moment. Sensing tension, Mom leaned in with graceful strength, and offered a gift—a completely unexpected message I'd needed for years:

"I love you, Sandy. Don't be ashamed of telling your stories—it's okay. What you remember is true. It was never your fault—it was mine. You were a sweet girl; hurt by the pain I caused. And you survived. Now, tell your story. Make it our story. Talk about it now because it won't exist when you come Home.

She hugged and kissed me, said "I love you," and disappeared.

All the while, Jesus reclined beside me, peaceful, present, eyes closed—offering steady love that asked nothing in return. He invited me to stay awhile and rest.

"Today when you hear his voice, don't harden your hearts." So there is a special rest still waiting for the people of God. So let us do our best to enter that rest. Hebrews 4:11, NLT.

LOVE TALK   Sandy

17

ETERNAL DREAMS

He uncovers mysteries hidden in darkness;
he brings light to the deepest gloom.
Job 12:22, NLT

Six months after Nathan relocated to heaven, I found myself overcome by a heavy, unshakable sense of impending sorrow. His first birthday away from us was drawing near, and with it came a deep dread—not only of that day, but of other holidays and traditions we once shared.

Grief, in its rawest form, doesn't just touch the heart—it envelops the entire body. On the night of September 6th, I slipped into bed, curling beneath the covers like a frightened child seeking refuge. I pressed in close to my husband, John, our arms encircling my shattered heart. The weeping continued until sleep finally brought relief.

Sometime around 3 a.m., I suddenly awoke—but not in my bedroom. I was alert, yet somehow elsewhere, alive in a place that felt outside of time. Even now, it's hard to put into words. It was as if I had stepped into a hidden dimension where holy presence breathed beauty and goodness. In this place I witnessed a sacred mystery:

> My husband, John, and I are walking hand in hand along a cedar path, through an expansive park-like setting. Soft green rolling hills stretch in every direction as far as our eyes can see. Immense trees of exceptional height tower above us like iconic skyscrapers. Limbs draped in vibrant foliage, twist and curl in the shape of a massive archway over the path we're on.
>
> Off in the far distance, hundreds of folks are milling around and celebrating in a recreation area that looks like a miniature model. Colorful fireworks pop and sparkle, sprinkling glitter across the sky above, broadcasting the party below.
>
> In an instant the scene changes, like when a camera zooms in on a specific object. John and I are walking the cedar path, but distant views vanish and everything around us appears close, as in real-time.
>
> Off to our left is a round wooden picnic table filled with high-school boys, sitting shoulder to shoulder around the circle. I can't hear their conversation, but their laughter and gestures speak of fond friendship and fun.
>
> The boy on the far side of the table, facing our direction, notices us walking past them. He suddenly stands up, waves his arms wildly, and shouts with great enthusiasm, "Hey! Hey! We found him! We found Nathan! We found Nathan!"
>
> The boy sitting directly across from him, with his back to us, turned around toward us. Much to my astonishment, it was

Nathan! He looked me straight in the eyes, his face beaming, and joyfully shouted, "Hi Mom! I'm alive! I'm alive!" Every cell in my body recognized his voice and I was astounded by the perfect clarity of his speech!

In this world, Nathan was unable to articulate most words because of severe apraxia.[238] One of Nathan's most difficult struggles was having words in his heart that he could not say. It was hard for us, too. We desperately wanted to hear Nathan's thoughts and feelings. I suppose our parental yearnings were merely a hint of the ache God feels when you and I go through our days not sharing our minds and hearts with him.

As quickly as Nathan's words left his lips, he happily turned back toward his buddies, content to pick up where he left off, and I startled awake.

"NO! I don't want to wake up! Go back!" I cried without a sound, "I want to be with Nathan!"

But there was no going back.

I slipped out of bed to record the dream in my journal, wanting to remember every single captivating feature.

Grief is tricky. It can trigger memories that you want to forget, and muddle matters you want to remember. I wasn't about to let this encounter escape full recognition.

The boy who waved his arms, shouting ecstatically, "We found him! We found Nathan!" left me baffled.

Over the years, I've learned the benefits of pausing to ask God questions when reality doesn't seem to match my grid. Honest Love Talks have led to discoveries I never would have enjoyed had I simply leaned on my own limited understanding.

Tuned to the most pressing question within, I wondered aloud on paper: "Why did the boy say, 'We found him! We found Nathan!' Do kids get lost in heaven?"

You need a bit of backstory here to understand why my train of thought automatically traveled in this direction. It's tied to the tangible neural map in my brain.

When Nathan was four-years-old we affectionately referred to him as our unguided missile. Self-propelled and fueled by an independent streak, he bolted from our home through the neighborhood and bordering forested greenspace. As far as he was concerned, the escapades were innocent, exciting adventures. People tell us Nathan came by his pioneer spirit naturally.

There was something mysterious and alluring to Nathan about an unlocked door into a neighbor's house. I can't remember all the DVDs, cameras, and other gadgets we discovered under Nathan's bed and sheepishly had to return. Wasn't it Mother Theresa who said, we learn humility by humiliation? I believe she was right. Nathan always told us exactly where he found his treasures and willingly apologized to the rightful owners.

I lost count of the number of times our family, friends, and the local police formed search parties to help us look for our missing boy. Those hunts held some of the scariest moments of my life. "We found him!" was a familiar phrase every fiber of my being knew fully, in a different time and place.

That's why I was puzzled. I wanted to know why the boys were looking for Nathan.

When I finished placing the dot under the question mark in my journal, a flow of words passed through my mind: *They wanted to find the boy (Nathan) who brought Me great glory.*

I sat stunned in a dim haze of eternal mystery.

My mind drifted back to those countless letters and heartfelt messages from high-school students who gathered around their school flagpoles, praying earnestly for Nathan in a city more known for its agnosticism and intellectual doubt than for faith. I thought of the little children in grade school who, after hearing of Nathan's accident, sent us drawings—innocent, tender pictures of their conversations with God. I remembered the 20-year-old woman who, for the first time in her life, saw the faces of her loved ones through the gift of Nathan's corneas. And then there was the grandfather whose life was quietly slipping away, now laughing and playing with his grandchildren again. Nathan's kidney had given him a second chance.

More than 3,000 people packed into a standing-room-only crowd to honor Nathan at his Celebration of Life. During the open mic, person after person stood, voices trembling with emotion, to share stories of how Nathan, our special young man with Down syndrome, had quietly and profoundly shaped their lives. It became unmistakably clear: Nathan's short time on earth had sent out ripples of eternal significance, reaching farther than we had ever imagined.

On the gloomy night before his seventeenth birthday, I was teetering on the outermost edge of my coping abilities. In a moment of transcendence, Love ventured into my dreams filling my senses with boundless goodness, and timeless clarity. I was creatively drawn into a new way of seeing, thinking, and feeling about Nathan, where fear began to loosen its grip and the stress-fractures in my heart slowly began to mend.

Grief continued to be a fierce force to be reckoned with, but its hold on me was noticeably different. My way of being had shifted.

I reveled in knowing that God doesn't stand at a distance from our pain. He steps right into it, with tenderness and power to reveal what is good, and beautiful, and to continue the deep work of making us whole. His desire for us is not just survival or coping—it's restoration. Even in the shadowed valleys of death, there are seeds of life waiting to break through. There, too, we are invited to grow, and flourish.

So when you finally crawl into bed, worn and weary, take heart. No place in your soul is too barren, too broken, or too far gone. Even while you sleep God draws near and continues to quietly mend what you think is beyond repair.[239]

You are going to be okay.

God works the night shift.[240]

An Invitation to Action

1. Invite God to speak to you in whatever way that He wants, including while you sleep.

2. Record what you can recall of any vivid dreams you experience in your journal.

3. Ask God if there's anything He wants you to understand about the dream, and write down whatever comes to mind. If He wants to give you insight, He absolutely can and will. If nothing comes right away, don't worry—just stay open and attentive. It's the Holy Spirit's role to bring clarity in His time. Like anything, discernment grows with practice.[241]

18

MYSTERY ON HEAVEN'S DOORSTEP

Miracles are signs, and like all signs, they are never about themselves; they're about whatever they are pointing toward. Miracles point to something beyond themselves. But to what? To God himself. That's the point of miracles—to point us beyond our world to another world.

Eric Metaxas

On January 24th, my mom experienced her final awakening. She left this world for a new life that you and I can only imagine in our wildest dreams.

Being with a loved one who is about to enter eternity is wrapped in wonder. I had a front-row seat watching mysteries unfold during Mom's final days with us.

Mom had a habit of re-positioning the Mickey Mouse watch she wore on her left wrist. For over 30 years, that favorite time-teller traveled the world with her. Even though she could have worn something far more *fancy*, Mom liked Mickey. His big hands pointed to large numbers, friendly to tired eyes.

Each morning, without fail, Mom wound her watch nine times to keep it from skipping a beat. When leather bands wore out, new ones took over keeping Mickey close through the years.

On Mom's graduation day, much to our astonishment, Mickey had a surprise for all of us which I noted in my journal.

Journal Entry January 24th—Mom Goes Home

Mom lies peacefully, unresponsive for hours. According to the hospice nurse, her departure is close.

Our family surrounds Mom, making our best effort to sing *The Battle Hymn of the Republic*, the graduation song Mom requested a few days earlier. Bumbling through our tears, we choke out the melody:

> "Mine eyes have seen the glory of the coming of the Lord. He is trampling out the vintage where the grapes of wrath are stored. He hath loosed the fateful lightning of His terrible swift sword, His truth is marching on. Glory, glory hallelujah…. Glory, glory hallelujah…"

In the middle of that glory-glory chorus, Mom's eyes suddenly open wide, the size of quarters, startling all of us. Rallying every ounce of strength left in her weary body, she fixates on something above and beyond her. We all look, too. None of us know what she sees *up there*, but whatever it is, keeps her spellbound through several slow deep breaths. Then she squints, like you do when the sun is too bright for your eyes, closes her lids tightly, and leaves us.

We're all stunned.

Looking at my sister Kelly, a medical expert and former critical care nurse, I ask, "Kelly, have you ever seen anything like that before?"

"I've seen many people pass, but nothing like that!" she replied, shaking her head no.

Keeping standard protocol, Kelly checks the clock and announces, "Time of death is 3:44 pm."

Meagan, the hospice nurse arrives shortly thereafter, takes Mom's vitals, confirms Mom's passing, and says, "Time of death is 4:12 pm."

Kelly clarifies, "Meagan, Mom passed at 3:44 pm."

Meagan nods in agreement, logs the time, and signs the official papers.

We remove Mom's jewelry. Dad places it on their bedroom dresser, and we do the best we can to comfort one another.

* * *

It's 10 pm. All of us are weary, hoping sleep will bring relief.

Dad walks out of his bedroom, hands Kelly Mom's watch, and says, "I'd like you to take Mom's Mickey Mouse watch home to Rachael (Kelly's youngest daughter who is autistic). I think she'll like it." Wiping tears from her cheeks, Kelly receives the gift with gratitude and a warm hug.

Looking at the watch, Kelly's jaw suddenly drops open in shock. Her eyes nearly pop out of her head as she exclaims, "Oh, my stars! You're not going to believe it! Look at this!"

Turning the watch toward us, the room falls silent.

Mickey's hands are frozen at exactly 3:44 p.m.—the very moment Mom took her final breath, the instant she finished her race and stepped into life ever after.

We stare together stunned, suspended in sacred mystery. The God of all comfort captures our hearts by confounding our minds.

I'm undone by the sheer wonder of it all.

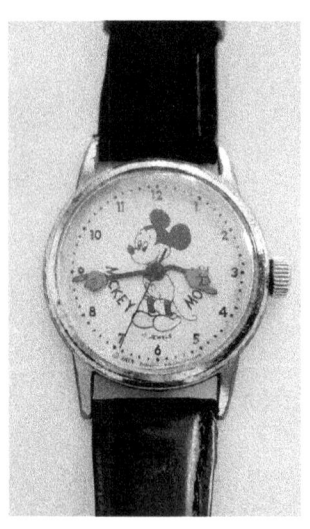

Years later, while enjoying a hot shower, my thoughts floated back to the day Mom passed, and the astonishment we all felt over her watch stopping with her final breath. I knew it wasn't simply a coincidence, and I kept wondering if I had missed something.

Was there more to this mystery than I understood?

With warm water pouring over my head, I looked up and whispered, "God, is there something more you want me to know about Mom's watch stopping when it did?"

Almost instantly, a gentle thought rose to the surface:

"Your times are in My hands."

The words resonated, full of peace and promise.

It was an echo of hope gently rolling from God's heart to mine; a mirror image of God's life within, reflecting the very words I had often whispered in my darkest moments: "My times are in your hands."[242]

As we live this life, in the tension of the already and not yet, we all need someone to help us shoulder our grief and gently guide us toward meaning. So, I invite you to raise your voice to heaven and wait. Listen for an echo. Stay tuned-in for Love to speak. Mysteries are yet to be encountered.

Your best whispers are yet to be heard – whispers designed to bring renewal, fulfillment, and joy.

Why? Because you were created for conversation with God. And your healing matters – not only for you, but for those you love, and the sake of the common good.[243]

An Invitation to Action

1. Has a mystery ever captured your heart with awe? Make a note in your journal about that unexplainable event, and what your thoughts were about God's possible involvement at the time.

2. Ask one or two good friends if they have ever experienced something they couldn't explain, that they thought might be supernatural. Write a brief summary of what they share with you in your journal.

3. On a scale of one to ten, how easy is it for you to believe that miracles happen today? What has contributed to this perspective?

19

CHOCOLATE CHIP COOKIES?

Nothing in life is to be feared, it is only to be understood.
Now is the time to understand more, so that we may fear less.

Marie Curie, physicist and first woman to win a Nobel prize

"Mary, I have a question for you: Can you imagine yourself in the kitchen following the steps in a recipe to make chocolate chip cookies?"

Cracking a smile she replied, "Yes."

"OK. How are you able to do that?" I asked.

"Well... It's not magic. I just see it in my mind," she answered.

"Exactly! You can picture it in your mind because God designed you with an imagination. You have an innate ability to perceive mental images, ideas, and sensations based on what you've learned and experienced. If your nose catches a whiff of fried bacon wafting through the room, what comes to mind?"

"Bacon."

"Yes. When you read text, hear words, or detect something with your five senses, your mind automatically creates a mental picture or concept attached to emotion and memory. It's simply how our Creator hard-wired us," I explained.

* * *

Albert Einstein said it well, "Your imagination is your preview of life's coming attractions. Logic will get you from A to Z; imagination will get you everywhere."

Imagination is essential to a meaningful life. It enables you to step outside your daily routine and daydream about travel, food, future plans, and new possibilities. It sparks hope, relieves boredom, eases pain, enhances pleasure, and enriches your most intimate relationships.[244]

That includes your relationship with God.

What we imagine when we think about God is profoundly important. In fact, we naturally move in the direction of our mental image of Him.[245] So, it's worth asking: *What is my image of God? Where did it come from? How was it shaped? What emotions are tied to it? And how can I know if it's accurate?* These are questions worth exploring with care.

Here's the simple point I'm pressing toward: our imagination plays a vital role in growing closer to God and experiencing healing.

After any kind of loss, it's important to pause and reflect: *Are we asking God to awaken our imagination so we can better understand who He is, what He's doing, and who He wants to be for us right now?* Are we becoming more aware of how He is at work in and around us? Are we asking for spiritual eyes and ears—to notice the meaningful ways He's revealing Himself?

If not, why not?

If we truly long to know the love of God more deeply, are we willing to make space—for the power, mystery, and leading of the Holy Spirit to shape our imagination and transform how we encounter God?

Ruth Burrows so beautifully said, "Prayer has far more to do with what God wants to do in us than with our trying to 'reach' or 'realize' or 'entertain' God in prayer. We can be quite certain that if we give the time to prayer, *God is always successful and that is what matters.*"[246]

There is never a moment when divine Love is not at work.[247]

Love always desires to communicate Its Self to us. This is God's irrevocable will and purpose. It's the reason why each one of us exists. The logical consequence for us must surely be to let ourselves be loved, to be there for Love to love us, to let ourselves be given to, let ourselves be worked upon by this great God and made capable of total union with Him.[248]

Imagine the possibilities. Who might we become if we practiced making space to be love-lavished by the transforming goodness of God?[249] [250] [251]

* * *

After raising four children and becoming a grandmother to eight, Mary reached a stage in life where she was ready to confront long-standing personal struggles. She was determined to focus her energy on emotional healing and *to do the inner work* necessary. Mary wanted to deal with damaging experiences from her past—injuries that had stolen her sense of freedom and joy[252]—so she could fully embrace her golden years and leave behind a meaningful legacy of love.

Mary had long avoided the painful parts of her life, but healing began the moment she reached out and brought her story into the light of God's love. A glimpse of a new beginning came when Mary turned toward God and began to speak honestly about what was weighing on her heart. My words appear in italics; Mary's are in regular font.

Mary, let's begin with a few deep cleansing breaths to calm your body and mind. Inhale peace, and exhale any stress you're holding. Allow your body to completely relax. Continue to breathe deeply, releasing tension from each part of your body. Notice every area starting with your head and slowly moving to your toes. With each breath, release any tension and relax a little bit more.[253]

We silence any voice that is not in complete alignment with Perfect Love.

Mary, fix your thoughts on God and let's ask for divine guidance and wisdom.[254]

Lord, you are the One who created Mary. You were with her the moment she was conceived in her mother's womb. You were with her through her childhood and adulthood, right up to this specific moment in time. You are here with her now. We ask You to reveal Yourself to Mary in whatever way she needs for a fresh start in her healing process.

Lord, grace us with spiritual awareness. Open our eyes and ears to the truth of who You are, our Ultimate Reality. Help us to know You more fully, to sense Your heart, and to rest in Your thoughts. We open ourselves to receive every expression of love You have for Mary today. Amen.

Mary, your Creator designed magnificent places on earth for you to enjoy. You've already traveled to areas that you long to revisit. Now, imagine yourself in one of those beautiful spots and relax from head to toe. Let peace settle over you. With the senses God has given you, take in the colors, the light, the sounds. Notice the details around you. Breathe deeply and take it all in. Simply be there.

You're completely safe and secure, immersed in God's love,

Can you describe the place for me?

"I'm snorkeling in Hawaii, surrounded by blues and greens and yellows. I see myself in the blue water, moving in the motion of the waves. The water doesn't feel warm or cold, just comfortable."

Where is God in the picture?

"In the water on my left."

God is with you. He is always with you and he loves being with you, Mary. He's very aware of the burden you're carrying. It's too heavy for you and he wants to help you. Do you notice God doing anything?

"No. I don't really notice anything."

Ahh. This is a sweet time. God is simply here to be with you, to love you. What else comes to your awareness?

"He's standing in the water. We're not very far from shore."

"Yes."

"We're hugging. We're standing on the shore together. He's next to me on my left."

Where is God looking?

"I don't know."

OK. Can you turn toward God and simply notice where he's looking?

"He's looking at me."

Is there anything else you notice?

"He's sort of smiling. . .I guess."

Okay. You've been carrying a heavy burden. What does it look like?

"A BIG boulder."

What does it feel like?

"It's very, very heavy… like a ton of weight."

How has the burden affected you?

"It's taken a lot of energy and worn me out. I get easily discouraged."

Mary, a ton is two thousand pounds. That's way too heavy for one person. Do you want to ask God to help you give that burden to Him?

"Yes."

Are you giving your burden to God?

"Yes."

What does He do with the burden?

"I don't see anything. (pause) . . . I know what the answer is supposed to be…"

OK. Let's take a moment to pause and breathe deeply—take a slow, cleansing breath and allow your body to relax. There's no pressure in this place. There isn't "one right" answer, and there is no "supposed to" here. You are safe in God's love and peace.

You don't have to figure anything out. Just rest, and let yourself be gently led. The Holy Spirit is tender and creative, always working with kindness to brings healing.

Lord, we ask You now—Please show Mary what You want her to know about the burden she gave to You.

"I see Jesus with his hands lifted high and wide, and the burden towers over Him. The boulder is really tall compared to Him. That's all I see."

The boulder appears huge and towers over Jesus?

"Yes."

Ok. Lord, what do You want us to understand?

"I know the answer. The boulder is only huge from my point of view."

Yes, Mary. And I sense God's deep compassion for you. He truly understands how heavy this burden feels in your everyday life—especially because your love for your children and grandchildren runs so deep.

I wonder… is there a part of you that's unsure if God is really big enough to carry this for you? Are you quietly worried that maybe it's too much—even for God?

"Yeah …deep sigh… I guess I do."

I understand—you are deeply devoted to your family, and you've been carrying this burden for such a long time. It makes sense that it feels so heavy.

Let's ask for His perspective. Lord, how do You see Mary's burden?

"Nothing comes to mind."

That's OK. Listening to God is a skill that grows with practice over time. That's why relationships and community are important. We learn and heal best with others. It's how God made us. May I tell you what I see?

"Sure!"

When we asked God for His perspective, the boulder towering over Jesus shrunk down to a small blue-green marble in the palm of His hand. He was playing with it in His palm, rolling it around, noticing the colorful swirls inside the marble.

"But … this burden is too serious for me to imagine God playing with it!"

I understand what you're saying. It's a curious picture, isn't it? But what I sense is not dismissal—it's a holy good-hearted delight. Creation, after all, began in joy. And even now, God's creativity is playful and purposeful. He created you and your family in love, and delights in the intricate design of each life.

He sees your burden fully—and He sees beyond it. He loves your children, and their children even more than you do. And He is with them, actively reaching out and pursuing them with good intentions.[255]

"But…when my kids were little, I didn't know anything about depression and I yelled at my kids. I had a lot of anger. I can't help but think that I hurt them and turned them away."

That's a valid concern, Mary. God is revealing something important to you. Part of the burden you're carrying over your children is guilt and shame. It sounds like you're blaming yourself, thinking that some of their choices are because you yelled and weren't a good enough mom. You believe that somehow, you're responsible. Am I hearing that right?

"Yes. Mark and I loved them and gave them so many more opportunities than we had as kids. But… I was a yeller and made a lot of mistakes."

I understand, Mary. Let's ask God for wisdom. God, will you show us the truth about the guilt and shame that Mary is carrying so that she can heal? (Long pause)

"I can't see anything."

It's OK Mary. A picture comes to my mind.

I see you standing at the foot of the cross, looking up at Jesus as He hangs there. Can you imagine yourself in that place?

"Yes."

Now, look down around the base of the cross. Notice the drops of blood that have fallen from the wounds of Jesus. This is visible evidence of His deep, personal love for you.

Jesus gave His life to free you from the weight of condemnation, from guilt over your mistakes, especially the "mom guilt" you've carried so long.

Can you see the drops of blood there at the bottom of the cross?

"Yes."

Mary, that blood—His blood—is your life source. It holds the power to release you, to renew you, to make you whole.[257]

Now, gently lift your eyes. Can you see Jesus on the cross above you?

"Yes"

Let yourself linger there a moment. This is holy ground. You have his complete attention now. His loving eyes are fixed on you. He feels your heartache over your children. He's in your pain with you and doesn't want you to carry it alone anymore.

Take a moment now and open your hands in a posture of surrender.

Picture your hands holding the guilt, shame, regret, and heaviness you've been carrying for years.

Now, lift it all up to Jesus and see Him receive everything you release.

Watch as He takes it into Himself—into His body.

See your wrongs, your anger, your past mistakes being drawn into His wounds.

They don't remain with you—they dissolve into Him, completely absorbed.

Release every failure and regret. Let it all flow into Jesus. Watch it disappear into His body, fading from sight.

Stay in this moment as long as you need and release everything related to that burden. There's no rush. Notice the weight lifting as Jesus takes it from you one portion at a time. Let me know when everything is released and you're ready to continue.

"I'm done."

Take a few deep breaths now, and tune in to your body. Notice what is different. The burdens aren't yours anymore. You are free.[258] *Mary, what are you sensing?*

"Something shifted".

Yes. I sense the shift, too. Is there anything else you want to leave at the cross now?

I don't think so. That was the big one.

OK. Let's ask God for wisdom. God, lead us. What else do you want Mary to know?

"Hmm . . . I see eyes."

And what do the eyes mean?

"He sees! He sees everything!"[259]

Yes. That is true. Lord, what is important for Mary to understand about this?

"He sees me. He really sees me! He sees everything about me. He knows exactly what I'm going through. He knows about all that I've been through. He knows everything... all of it!"

Yes, it's true. God sees you. He sees the burden you gave Him, and He has treasures for you.[260] *Are you open to receiving a gift in exchange for your guilt?*

"Yes!"

Remember when you were standing with Jesus on the sandy seashore in Hawaii?

"Yes."

Let's go back to that lovely place. Take a few deep breaths and let yourself settle into the beauty around you once again. Notice the blues in the water and sky above. Try to tune in to the warmth of the sun and the gentle breeze on your skin. See the soft movements in the water in front of you. Are you on the seashore next to Jesus, like you were earlier?

"Yes."

God has a gift for you, a tangible symbol to replace the boulder you gave him. When you're ready, turn toward him and tell me what you notice?

"I don't notice anything."

It's OK. Your honesty is priceless. Always say what is true. This brings freedom. God, what gift do you have for Mary today? (pause) Mary, do you sense anything?

"No."

It's OK. That's why we listen to God together. He teaches us how to hear and perceive as we practice in relationship with others. May I share what I see?

"Yes!"

I see Jesus placing that blue and green marble into your hand -- the same one He had been playfully rolling around in His palm earlier. I believe it's a sacred reminder: He sees it all—everything about you, your children, your grandchildren. And He holds each of you tenderly and firmly in the palm of His hand.[261]

There is nothing strong enough to pull your family from His grasp.[262]

Nothing at all can separate you from His Perfect Love.[263]

Right now, even as you listen, His goodness is quietly and faithfully pursuing your children every hour of every day, surrounding them in ways you may not yet see.[264] Mary, is anything else coming to your awareness?

"I see eyes again." Beautiful. God is amplifying His point. Scripture says, "The eyes of the Lord search the whole earth in order to strengthen those whose hearts are fully committed to Him."[265]

God is doing that right now—strengthening you with reassurance. He sees your beautiful, faithful heart. He knows the depth of your devotion. And He wants you to remember that you were personally chosen by Him to be the mother of your children, and the grandmother of theirs.

He entrusted these lives to you not by accident, but with purpose. And as much as you love them—God loves them even more. Their well-being is not beyond Him. It's not too complicated, or too far gone. It's not too heavy for God.

In fact, He delights in pouring out His goodness on them. You can count on Him to show up for them, again and again, in the ways they need most.

And Mary, right now, God is here for you. He sees every part of your heart, even the places you keep tucked away. He understands the swirl of emotions—the concern, the confusion, the longings. Even when it feels like nothing is changing, nothing is moving, God is at work quietly and powerfully—in you.

He hears your prayers. Every single one. To Him, they rise like sweet perfume—shifting the atmosphere, inviting heaven into earth.

So, keep praying for your children. But do it now with a lighter heart. You don't have to carry it all. God is doing the heavy lifting. And He will never, ever let go.

Mary, that massive, one-ton burden is no longer yours to carry.[266] *You've handed it over and now, you're free to live in peace and joy.*[267]

You exchanged that heavy weight for something much lighter and more beautiful. The blue-green marble held in God's hand, is now yours.

Take a moment to soak in God's love. Ask God to fill every part of you—every cell in your body.

And let the marble be your reminder: You're not alone in this struggle. You are partnering with Almighty God for the good of your family. You can live freely and lightly, caring for them with God.

Mary, is there anything else on your mind?

"Yes. I want to thank God for what He's done. . . Lord, thank you for the marble and for showing me Your perspective. Thank You for seeing me. Thank You for seeing my love for my family. Thank You for taking my burden . . .I can't say thank you enough."

Yes, Lord. We pause now to honor You. Thank you for who You are. Your redeeming love leaves us in awe. Thank you for giving us the grace to see and hear what You are saying. Thank You for sharing your good gifts with Mary.[268] *Thank You for helping Mary view her reality according to Your ultimate reality. Would you imprint Mary's body, soul, and spirit with the truth and write it deeply in her heart.*[269]

Lord, let Mary's encounter with You be like a seed planted deeply in rich soil—one that takes root, grows strong, and bears lasting fruit in the days, and months to come. Continue to help Mary to listen and hear Your voice. May your whispers become ever clearer and more familiar. Show Mary how she can nurture her friendship with You so that it flourishes into a source of strength and great joy. Remind Mary often that she is held, guided, and deeply loved. May partnering with You become a defining quality of Mary's life.

We thank you for this time together with You, and close it now in Jesus name, amen."

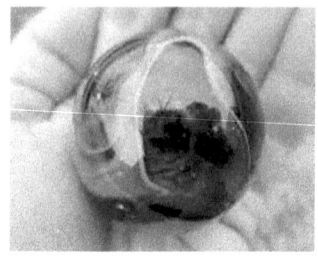

For the Kingdom of God is not a matter of what we eat or drink, but of living a life of goodness and peace and joy in the Holy Spirit.

Romans 14:17, NLT

I sit upon a checkered blanket in a meadow filled with lush, springy grass. Buttery sunlight touches the hair draped over my shoulders, carefree strands tickling my cheek.

Jesus sits next to me. He emanates incandescent light, Love reverberating through the air around me. His nearness is a warm hug, and tears roll down my cheeks.

"Hello," I whisper. "I'm so glad you're here. Thank you for being with me. I love You so much!"
I don't know what else to say.

Jesus smiles, the corners of His eyes crinkling. His compassion floods my being. I may be without words, but here in His presence I am never without a home.

I look down at the bundle of books in my hands. Their covers entice with magical designs, but the insides feel dark, flat, and captivating, like sinking quicksand.

"I'm sad to show you these. But, then again, you already know. I've decided I don't want them anymore."

Before completing my thought, Jesus extends His strong hand to lift the weight off of me. The books vanish like mist in His grasp, and a writing pen appears in His palm.

"Someday, you will hold a stack of your own books," He whispers. "The stories we will write together."

His words take my breath away. I can barely reply, "Ohh, Thank you!"

A tiny seed of new life takes root, fresh confidence secured by His word.

I pick up the pen and start to write a new story—one co-created with the Author of life.

LOVE TALK

Jenny

20

THERE'S NO PLACE LIKE HOME

> *Every time you listen with great attentiveness to the voice that calls you the Beloved, you will discover within yourself a desire to hear that voice longer and more deeply. It's like discovering a well in the desert. Once you have touched wet ground, you want to dig deeper.*
>
> *Henri Nouwen*

They say, "Home is where your heart is," but what do *they* know anyway?

What if your early years were lived in an unsheltered place of awkward disconnections, where belonging and affection unraveled? What if the tender essence of your substance and promise went unnoticed or was treated harshly in the dwelling you called home?

Amanda didn't want her daddy to leave. She didn't ask to be abandoned. And she didn't sign up to parent her younger siblings from the time she was six years old. She simply stepped in because everyone else stepped out. In subtle, unseen ways these experiences became deeply imprinted in her memory.

Fast forward forty years. Amanda had forgiven her parent's mistakes more times than she could count. Little by little, as she was ready, she dismantled the ghost structures of old realities and carefully tended to her hidden heart wounds.

One day she mentioned hitting an impasse. The lost lonesome little girl within was burdened,[270] longing to feel at home in God's love. Years of ongoing struggle had set the stage for battles with anxiety and confusion about her worth:

> *I desperately want to know God as my loving heavenly Father, but I just can't get there. There's a disconnect. This longing has been with me for decades. I don't know what's in my way or how to break through. I love Jesus with all of my heart. He is my Lord and friend. The Holy Spirit is my daily Companion, Helper, and Counselor.*
>
> *It makes no sense. I can easily honor God as the King of Kings who rules from His heavenly throne, but I'm missing something. I just can't connect with God's fatherly affection. I want to experience God as my tender Father.*[271] [272]
>
> *My mind believes that God sees everything about me*[273] *and that He cherishes me as his special girl,*[274] *but I want to know God as my loving Daddy.*[275]

Right up-front Amanda defined the issue she wanted to explore together. But before proceeding, she shared a write-up from her journal about a surprising incident that happened a few days earlier:

In the morning, I decided to switch up my usual walking route. Instead of meeting at the high school, I texted my friends, "Let's start from Amy's house and walk to the coffee shop." Everyone agreed, and we set off.

At the first intersection, we paused to decide: Shall we take the flat, easy path or the hillier, more challenging one? We chose the hill—wanting a bit of a push before our coffee. After making the climb, we grabbed our drinks to go.

Since we were carrying hot coffee, I suggested we take the easier route back. Chatting among ourselves, we began walking toward Amy's house.

Suddenly, Amy shouted, "Hey, hold up you guys!"

I looked up and saw her—a tiny blonde-haired girl in a pink sundress, wearing a butterfly backpack over her shoulders. She couldn't have been more than three years old, and she was walking right down the middle of a busy street, completely unaware of the danger!

We moved in quickly and guided her safely off the road as cars zoomed by us. Scanning the area, we searched for any sign of an adult who might know her.

I called 911 while my friends, Jody and Amy, did their best to keep the energetic little girl from running back into the street. Each of us took on a different role, helping to comfort, distract, and keep her safe as we waited for the police to arrive.

As the officers approached, fear swept over the little girl's face, and she began to fidget anxiously. When one of them reached for her arm to keep her still, she panicked—crying uncontrollably and struggling to break free.

Instinctively, I scooped her up and held her close, trying to comfort her. I gently told her we were friends, and that we'd help her find her mommy and daddy. I promised to take her home.

My friend Amy told the officers she was confident the little girl could find her way home if we just gave her a chance. We offered to walk with her and keep her safe as she searched. The officers agreed and followed a short distance behind us.

As we walked, we stopped at each house and gently asked her, "Is this your home?"

Each time, she shook her head and said, "No."

Then we came to a house with a small bicycle in the driveway. Something about it caught her eye. She brightened, ran up the driveway, and tried to open a side garage door—but it was locked.

We encouraged the little girl to try the front door. She hurried that way, opened it easily, went inside, and closed the door behind her.

That's when the officers stepped in. They knocked, but there was no response. After a long wait, a tearful woman finally came to the door. She explained to the officers that she had been working from home, trying to manage her job while caring for her three young children. She hadn't realized, until moments ago, that her daughter had quietly slipped out and wandered away.

As Amy and I walked back to her house, cars sped past us, zipping through the very spot where the little girl had been standing earlier. I couldn't shake the feeling that her rescue had been divinely orchestrated.

It seemed our ordinary plans had been quietly rearranged and perfectly timed to guide this little girl safely back home.

Later that day, in a quiet moment of reflection, a new insight came to me.

It suddenly struck me—the blonde-haired, blue-eyed little girl was a reflection of me as a child. I saw my own innocence in her, and the helplessness I felt in the face of dangers I couldn't understand or control. Many of those dangers were beyond my awareness at the time, too.

As I sat with that realization, faces came to mind—people God had placed in my life to guide and protect me. Throughout my childhood, He had quietly surrounded me with helpers who stepped in to shield me from very real harm.

I'm not saying that the impact of childhood trauma hasn't been painful. It has. But even in that truth, I also see that my parents never meant to hurt me. They were caught in their own struggles, doing the best they could with limited understanding and resources.

* * *

When Amanda woke up that day, she never would have guessed that a simple, unplanned change in her walking routine would place her exactly where she needed to be. But . . . Love has a way of leading us, even when we're unaware.

Now, all is well. The little girl is safe, her mother is relieved, and three good friends involved in the encounter are filled with quiet gratitude—for the mystery of timing, the mercy of divine interruptions, and the joy of helping guide a little girl safely home where she belongs.

Amanda's story stirred something in me. I began to wonder what else God might be orchestrating behind the scenes. Could there be mysteries still unfolding—gifts she had yet to discover? Was her encounter with the little girl, along with the lingering impact of her own childhood trauma, somehow connected to the solution for the very struggle she mentioned to me?

I'm always struck by how life's most meaningful moments are often subtle—unspoken, unseen, or hidden just beyond our awareness. Sometimes we carry a sense of quiet knowing, without being able to explain why.

Neuroscientists tell us this kind of *gut feeling* often draws on what we've already lived through—what we've seen, sensed, learned, and felt—stored deep in long-term memory. It may not always be clear, but it's real. And sometimes, it can be one way God gently leads us toward healing and insight we didn't know we were ready for.

This kind of language might be new to you—it is for many people I talk with. So, let me simplify by explaining two main types of memory:

Implicit Memory

Our earliest memories, especially those from before age three or four, are *implicit*, meaning they're stored in the body and outside of conscious awareness. At that early age, the brain hasn't yet developed the ability to store memories in verbal, narrative form.

Implicit memories cannot be recalled on purpose. They're non-verbal, automatic, and show up as emotions, behaviors, or sensations. They're *felt* more than *remembered*. Skills like riding a bike or tying your shoes are good examples—you just *know* how, even after years without practice. Some call this "retention without remembering." Now catch this: Implicit memory tends to be stronger and longer-lasting than explicit memory.

Explicit Memory

Explicit memory involves information you can intentionally recall and describe. For example, remembering *who* helped you ride a bike or *where* that happened. These memories are verbal, conscious, and organized.

Most memories fall neatly into one of these two categories. But trauma is different.

Traumatic memories—regardless of age—are often stored *implicitly*. That's because when trauma happens, the brain is flooded with stress hormones like cortisol. This overload can shut down the part of the brain responsible for processing and storing memories in a logical, verbal way. Language often goes offline during trauma, leaving those memories jumbled, vague, or "silent." They don't form a clear story, but live in the body as emotion or tension.[276]

When those implicit trauma memories are triggered later in life, they don't feel like the past—they feel immediate, intense, and out of proportion to what's actually happening. There's no obvious link to the original wound, yet the emotional charge is very real.

So, what does all of this have to do with Amanda and her struggle to feel God's fatherly love?

Walk with me through this line of thought.

When Amanda shared her struggle to experience God's love, I began to wonder if implicit memories—unconscious, body-stored memories from childhood abuse—might be influencing her in ways she didn't fully understand. Could these body memories be interfering with her ability to *feel* the Father's love, even though she firmly *believed* it to be true?

For over forty years, Amanda had accepted that God loved her—but the truth remained distant, disconnected from her emotions and her body.

I also wondered if these same implicit memories shaped her instinctive response to the little girl's panic. When the officer grabbed the child's arm, Amanda said she reacted *without thinking*. She rushed in, scooped the girl into her arms, and held her close to soothe and protect her. It was automatic—deeply embodied. Others nearby responded differently, shaped by their own histories and instincts.

Perhaps the little girl's distress stirred something unspoken in Amanda that echoed her own childhood pain. Maybe it tapped into memories of being hurt by her father, or the overwhelming burden of caring for her younger siblings at just six years old. It seemed as though powerful forces were at work beneath the surface, shaping her response without her even realizing it.

And yet, alongside all of that, I couldn't help but sense a quiet, mysterious goodness at work. It was as if an ordinary walk, reshaped by a spur-of-the-moment decision, led Amanda into a divinely orchestrated moment, not only for a frightened three-year-old girl, but also for a grown woman with blond hair and blue eyes, both longing to find their way home.

Amanda and I decided to continue exploring these ideas together in conversation with God.

Amanda's comments are written in regular font, and mine are in italics.

Amanda began slow-paced belly breathing to calm her body and enhance her focus.[277] We invited the Holy Spirit to lead us into truth. I prayed: "Father, you have heard the cries of Amanda's heart. You know how she longs to more fully know You as her loving heavenly Father. By faith, she believes that you are her *abba*, daddy. She wants to experience Your love as her own truth.[278] We ask for wisdom. Will you please open our eyes and ears, speak to us, and show us what is needed for healing?"

I waited quietly and then Amanda began to describe a picture that came to her.

"From a bird's-eye view, I see myself walking through a blizzard. I'm moving forward through the storm, pressing on to reach the Lord—trying to find my place with Him. It's hard, but I'm determined to keep going."

And now?

"The scene shifted. Jesus is close beside me, walking with me. We're both facing forward, heading in the same direction."

Tune in to what you see, hear, smell, taste, and feel. What are you sensing?

"I hear the wind and feel the storm pushing hard against me. I don't feel peace or joy right now, but I feel a strong resolve. I'm determined to keep going with Jesus. Even in the storm I feel confident—like we can do this together."

What else do you notice?

"Jesus isn't untouched by the storm. He's not some spirit floating above it all—He's bundled up like me. He's right in the storm with me, feeling the same cold, the same wind. He's enduring it with me."

Do you have anything you'd like to ask Him?

"How much longer? Are we almost there?"

What comes to you?

"I see a picture of a warm, sunny paradise-like place just ahead. It's close."

"So, to clarify . . .the storm is behind you, and you're near the edge of something beautiful?"

"Yes. It's like I'm looking at a living image, split in two. On one side, Jesus and I are bundled up in the storm—it's dark, like dusk, and we're leaning into the wind. On the other side is blue sky, sunlight, white sand, and water—like a beautiful vacation spot. I'm standing near the edge in the middle, between the two images."

Is there anything keeping you from stepping into the sunny place?

"I don't know. I want to, but I hesitate. I don't know if it's OK. Should I wait? Or am I supposed to step across?"

Why don't you ask God?

"The words that come to me are: 'Not yet.' It's not time."

Ahhh. Very nice. You had an inner knowing that was cautioning you. Would you like to ask God to help you understand what that means?

"Yes... I see that I'm still in the storm, but the worst of it is behind me. The storm is not ahead of me anymore—it's behind me. And just ahead is a place of peace. I sense I'm close and a beautiful change is coming."

So, you're nearing the end of a long struggle, and what's ahead is safe and good?

"Yes."

Would you like to ask the Lord to confirm that you've heard correctly?

"Yes. I see myself in distress, crying out to God. I don't want false hope. I don't want to be disillusioned. I don't want the beautiful place I see to be like a mirage—something that looks real but disappears when I reach for it."

Beautiful! That's honest, Amanda. God always honors honesty. So Lord, we look to You. We silence any voice that's not from You. We want to know what is true about this place Amanda sees ahead.

"I sense reassurance that a blessing is coming that will carry me across the threshold—something that will move me into that peaceful place. It's not something I'm going to move into on my own. And it's not a vacation spot, or a temporary place to rest—it's more of a dwelling place, like a new season. A new era."

Where do you see your Heavenly Father in that new place?

"Hmmm...I looked and couldn't find Him at first. I tried to envision Him sitting on a throne, like I often do, but then I saw something different—He was in the water, playing, splashing, and laughing. He was having fun."

And where are you in the picture?

"At first, I was outside the scene. Then He invites me to come play with Him."

So, what do you do?

"I go right in! We're together in the ocean, leaning on floaties, holding hands, just talking. I feel relaxed and safe—like I belong. I'm an adult, as I am today, having a great conversation with Him. He's attentive, listening closely, offering wisdom. It seems like what a good father would do with a child he loves."

What else are you feeling?

"I feel very safe. I feel seen and treasured. There's no one else around and I have His full attention. I can tell He wants to be here with me. He's not distracted or trying to move on to someone else. He's happy to be together and wants to stay. That means so much to me."

Would you like to ask Him to help you receive more of His love, and to more easily trust?

"That question pricks something painful in my heart."

Can you name that pain?

"Yes. . . It's fear—fear of being rejected, and I see a picture of red and orange flames. I think they represent the pain."

What else is happening?

"Now there are blue flames beside the red and orange ones. The blue flames are God's love. The blue flames are consuming the other flames, slowly putting out the fire of my pain. God is showing me that I can trust His love more and more. The process is slow and steady, and He will continue to lead me."

Anything else?

"Yes. I feel close to something shifting, but I'm afraid I won't be able to step into it."

It's okay, Amanda. Perfect Love is holding your right now. He's providing you with a new sense of safety, belonging, and security. In your mind's eye, can you go with me to the foot of the cross and envision Jesus there with you?

"Yes"

Notice His body— the bloody wounds covering him. This is the evidence of God's burning love for you. His blood doesn't just cleanse you from sin—it heals you from the wounds caused by sin, including the sins of others.[279] By His wounds you have been healed.[280]

Would you like to offer your fear to Jesus?

"Yes."

Go ahead and lift your fear in your hands toward Jesus. Describe what you notice.

"My heart feels like a dark, heavy mass, bulky and weighted down. But when I lifted it up to Jesus, He reached down to me. As I opened my hands, He gently took over, lifting the burden out of them."

Beautiful. Now, notice how Jesus absorbs that heavy, dark mass into Himself. Watch as it disappears—fading completely into His body until it's gone. Can you see it?

"Yes. Its disappearing into Jesus. It's completely gone now."

Good. Now take a few deep, slow breaths. Inhale the breath of life, and as you exhale release the fear from your body. Tune in to what is happening with all of your senses. You're letting go of any residual fear, giving it all to Jesus. Notice the tension releasing. Notice the fear losing its grip and leaving your body like an empty vapor. Let me know when you sense a shift.

"It's gone now. I feel peace."

Take a moment now and rest in God's peace. Soak it in. Pay attention to how your body feels. Take a mental snap shot of how you're experiencing God in this moment, and ask God to help you integrate it in your memory. Enjoy this time basking in God's love. . .

Amanda when we release our fears to God he often offers a gift in exchange, to galvanize and empower us for the days ahead. Do you want to ask God if He has a gift for you --- a provision for you to receive?

"Ummm...I feel resistance coming up inside. I don't know why I'm resisting. I don't want to oppose what God has for me, but part of me is pulling back, hesitant.... I don't want to have false hope that He'll give me something I truly want—something unique that has special meaning to me. . . I just don't want to be disappointed."

I understand, Amanda. Your struggle is completely valid. You grew up in a home where what you needed and what you actually received were worlds apart. That gap is real, and it shaped you. Of course you feel hesitant. It's okay to bring that honestly to God. He already knows, and He welcomes you just as you are. You can be open with God about what's on your mind. Simply tell Him the truth.

"Lord, I want to be open to receiving all that You have for me, but I don't know if You want to give me something that I will like. I don't want to get my hopes up and then be disappointed. I want to know you as my loving daddy, and it's hard for me to trust."

Would you like to ask God to help you open up and receive what He has for you?

"Yes."

Go ahead do so, and describe what unfolds.

"When I cried out, Jesus moved around behind me to help me open my hands. His hands are around my hands and my hands are open. He placed something in my hand. The picture is so clear—I can't shake it! It looks like a snow globe. It's a round glass ball, with a house in the middle, surrounded by floating glitter."

What does the gift mean to you?

"It means, safety and security."

Yes! I sense that, too. The gift is a reminder that your sense of security, and belonging is best experienced dwelling in God's love. The glass globe says, "Amanda, you are home! You're right where you belong—embraced in the infinite love of Father, Son, and Holy Spirit.

"Yes! I know it! And it represents stability and grounding."

That's right. The kind that can carry you through any kind of storm.

Amanda, take a moment to notice how God's love has been showing up—like the glitter swirling inside your snow globe—in the recent scenes of your life. Your conversation with God just now beautifully mirrors your encounter with the three-year-old little girl earlier this week. That moment wasn't random. It was like a window into the spiritual realm—a visible sign of God's invisible grace.

When you crossed paths with her, your heart was instantly moved. You made that little girl a promise, offering your word that you would get her safely home.

"Oh, Wow! Yes, I did!"

That tenderness you felt for her, your deep, instinctive desire to protect and comfort, came from a sacred place within you. You scooped her up and held her close, not just to shield her from fear, but to communicate safety and love.

Can you bring that moment back to mind? Can you feel again how compassion surged through your body?

"Yes. I can!"

Stay there for a moment. Let yourself soak in that feeling. Let your whole being bathe in that love. That outpouring of compassion you had for her is only a glimpse—a fraction—of the overwhelming affection your heavenly Father feels for you.

Now, connect your deep compassion with God's perfect love for you. Sense His strong and tender arms around you, and how His adoration warms you from the inside out. You are held. You are loved. And you are home.

As you continue with your day, keep tuning your heart to the voice of Love—to the One who washes away your hurt and gently brings your longings into rhythm with His grace. Hear His tender whisper: "Come back soon… and stay a little longer."

Isn't it beautiful how the physical and spiritual often mirror each other?

"Wow! Yes! God is amazing!"

Take time this week to be still. Let yourself rest in the awareness of all you've experienced with God. Reflect on what you've seen, heard, and felt. Reflect on Scriptures that speak of His love, and the true home He offers.[281]

Linger. Listen closely. God has more to show you. Each time you release your heartache to Him and receive His grace, something in you is renewed—your heart, your mind, and your body are rewired with hope and healing.

Will you share with me what you discover next time we're together?

* * *

Amanda's renovation is ongoing, marked by increasing freedom and joy. Rather than replaying old narratives that once drove her to avoid her heavenly Father, she now runs to Him—raw, real, and just as she is. There is less striving to protect herself or to keep trouble at bay. Instead, she practices drawing close to God, finding safety and security at home in God's presence.[282]

So, what is Amanda's part in this remarkable post-trauma growth? What helps fuel her renewal in heart, soul, mind, and body?

Participation through intentional awareness and practice.

Amanda practices the *Reset*, tuning in with compassion to her inner world. She makes space for stillness—learning to release what no longer serves her, and to receive what she most needs in the shelter of Love's presence. In that sacred space, healing comes—not all at once, but steadily restoration and renewal happens.

Through her daily Love Talks with God, Amanda is keeping a quiet promise—to lovingly guide that precious blond-haired, blue-eyed little girl home. Home to where she's safe and secure.

Home to where loss is redeemed and all things are being made new.

An Invitation to Action

1. Looking back can offer fresh perspective, and inform you about how far you have come. Go back to the beginning of your journal notes and look specifically at where you were when you started. What differences do you see in yourself between then and now? Make a list in your journal of the obvious growth changes (the incremental wins) you've experienced.

2. Review your writings and identify the practices/tools that have empowered you to better understand and release your grief. Note how each practice has helped you.

3. Summarize how you plan to use these practices going forward.

A scene unfolds in prayer, revealing who I truly am.

Parents gather their children eager to see Jesus. The children in my class bubble with excitement. Yet, one small boy lingers sheepishly at the edge—reluctant and anxious. My heart aches for him. I want to coax him along, to share in this sacred occasion.

We walk single file along a gravel path, each step drawing me deeper into uncertainty that mirrors the reluctant boy's qualms. We find a grassy slope, I spread out a blanket, and arrange the children's gear. Jesus sits atop the gentle hill surrounded by joy.

Children climb over Him, giggles ringing out as they fiddle and tug at His beard. Jesus laughs in sheer delight. I feel at home—something I've longed for but never experienced with God. Parents engage Jesus in easy conversation with effortless smiles. I stand back in doubt, longing to belong yet terrified of stepping forward. Uncertainty screams, "Don't be a fool! Hope leads to humiliation. There's no for you room near Him."

I've been this way for too long. I can guide children to Jesus, but I can't seem to take myself.

"Go on, kids, hurry along!" Their longings grip me like a warm hug.

"Ms. Jackson, you're coming with us!" a boy cries out. His plea seizes my heart.

"No, no, it's okay. Run along, now. Today is especially for you. I'll stay here."

"We won't go without you, Ms. Jackson!" The reluctant child clasps my hand in fierce determination, his small fingers squeeze tightly, refusing to let go.

Anxiety consumes me. I'm not worried we'll be turned away. I'm afraid I'll be ignored, invisible - unworthy of notice. I don't know how to muster-up the faith.

A fragile thought surfaces: What if I take just one small step? Maybe, I'll find the strength to keep going. I don't want my shy little boy to miss out. With trembling resolve, I inch forward.

Instantly I find myself enveloped in Jesus's lap, my head against his chest. His heartbeat resonates through me in a rhythm that echoes inside and out. I'm wrapped in a cocoon of affection, a sanctuary I never knew existed. The world fades away as birds flap their wings and flowers dance in rhythm. Everything becomes one in this symphony of love.

Footsteps on the path tell me more children are coming. I must bring them to this Love like no other. They must know Him—especially the reluctant ones in the shadows, afraid to hope.

LOVE TALK

Susan J.

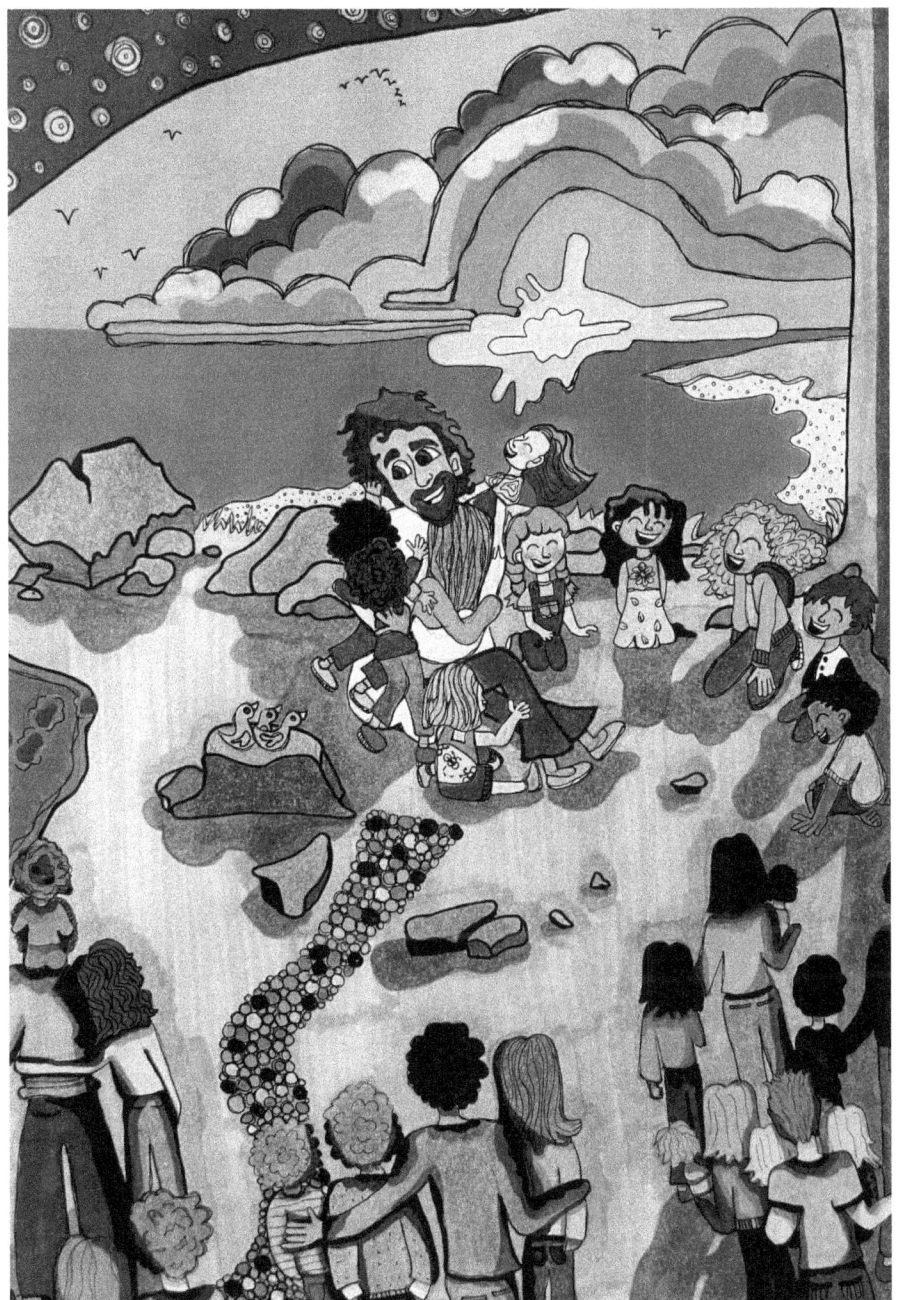

21

REDEEMING LOSS

You learn by practice. Practice over and over again in the face of all obstacles, some act of vision, of faith, of desire. Practice is a means of inviting the perfection desired. You are unique, and if that is not fulfilled, then something has been lost.[283]

Martha Graham, Mother of Contemporary Dance

Do you remember who you were when you first picked up this book? If you give it a moment's thought, I'll bet an answer will come to you.

Maybe you felt like you were drowning in grief, hoping for someone to throw you a lifeline after a death, a divorce, or a diagnosis that changed everything. Maybe you were dealing with rejection, cut off from someone you loved, stuck in the confusion and pain that comes with being shut out. Maybe you were just… alone. A friendship ended, a job disappeared, someone important moved on, or a beloved pet passed away—and suddenly you were left behind, disoriented, trying to make sense of it all.

If you're old enough to count your age in double digits, you've likely experienced many losses. By the time you close this book, I hope you have a better sense of why you feel and react the way you do, and how you think about the painful life-altering episodes in your story.

Loss creates unfamiliar, difficult terrain—far more complicated than most of us expect. It's messy, heavier and more taxing than most of us imagine. By now, I hope you realize something important: your grief is as unique as your fingerprint, your pain is real, your confusion is valid, and you are not broken or crazy.

I also pray that somewhere along the way, hope has crept back in. That you've started to believe—even just a little—that you, yes – you, *can* come out of heartbreak stronger and more resilient than you were before.

But know this: healing doesn't just happen. Good outcomes don't come simply because we hope for them. True transformation requires effort, intention, and the support of wise, steady companions. It's a journey—and one that's worth every step.

Since we all share the same human experience, bound by the same rhythms of life, loss, and love, this is worth saying again: *Healing and relationships go hand in hand.* They work together, side by side, in a powerful, creative partnership.

We heal best in connection with God, and with safe people who love us. We are not designed to do life alone. No one flourishes in isolation.

As a final step, I invite you to do something small but meaningful. Grab a pen, write this down, stick it on your mirror, and let it sink in:

How I choose to reflect on and tell my story affects my health and my relationships.

It's that simple—and that important.

Friend, an unrenewed mind causes damage within and without. When our stories remain unexamined, pain often leaks out in harmful ways. Left unresolved, it can seep out of us and into the lives of those we love—even generations yet to come.

But here's the good news: you're worth the work. And so are your loved ones.

Maybe that's why the Holy Spirit moved Jeremiah—the weeping prophet—to write these words:

"Listen, you women, to the words of the Lord; open your ears to what He has to say. Teach your daughters to wail; teach one another how to lament."

Teach one another how to lament. There is power in those words.

The best way to teach anything is by modeling – to live your message out loud. Use words to name what's going on inside you. Let your emotions be seen and expressed. Let the tears come. Feeling is healing.

Practice it. Live it. Be intentional. Do it for your own freedom, and for the ones you love. Do it for the little ones who haven't arrived yet—but who will one day inherit the atmosphere you help create.

The best gift you can give your family is your transforming self.[284]

And the journey begins with telling the truth—gently, honestly, and in love.

The stage is set for you to move forward on the healing path where losses are redeemed. I recall a conversation with Ashley, a young mom who lost her seven-year-old daughter, Emily, in a car accident. I'll never forget how God tenderly reached into Ashley's darkest despair and made a way where there wasn't one. Home alone with no one else to help, God showed up.

Ashley said, "There were times when I walked through the house and heard Emily call out to me from her room, from the hallway, or from the kitchen saying, 'Mom! I'm in here!' I felt like I was losing my mind! After weeks of this, I fell on my knees sobbing hysterically and screamed, 'God, I can't take it anymore. I can't live like this! Emily wasn't supposed to die before me!'[285]

A gentle voice interrupted me. *Ashley, give me your grief and I will redeem it.* I did not know what that meant, but it sounded better than being trapped in torment.

My thoughts were jumbled. I wasn't able to concentrate on anything for more than a few minutes. I started writing letters to God to help me focus and stay on task. In desperation, I spilled out my heart on paper in the morning, in the evening, and whenever I could grab ten minutes alone.[286]

My grief was messy. It looked different from one day to the next, changing temperature between morning, afternoon, and night. Anger, sadness, fear, guilt, hopelessness, shame, rage, resentment, self-pity, envy, hate, and thoughts of suicide surfaced up and out. Telling God everything helped me release the pain.[287]

I began to see waves of grief as an invitation from God for more inner healing. It's hard to put into words, but I feel tangibly different after I write to God. I'm lighter and can breathe easier. It's like the fresh, clean feeling after a long hot shower.

Sometimes, I sense God close to me, and other times, I don't. Buy it's okay. I believe God is with me, even in the brain fog. My goal is to stick with the process until I'm whole. So, I keep clinging to God, writing letters, releasing my grief, and receiving what He gives."[288] [289]

Today, Ashley is free of mental torment, and making good progress in recovery. Healing is incremental and steady. Love Talks, her go-to tool, are strategically therapeutic. Ashley shows up each morning with an honest, open, and willing heart. Embraced in everlasting arms, she is empowered, sustained, and carefully led to new vistas.

Ashley's tenacity to persist in caring for her heart wounds reminds me of a helpful prompt I learned from my friend, Jenny Donnelly. Using the word *REST* as an acrostic, Jenny highlights a way to find relief and peace:[290]

R - Release

E - Every

S - Single

T - Thing

Using the same acrostic, I like to combine Jenny's tip with another practice that promotes heart-soul-mind-body renewal. Paired together, I see them as two sides of the same coin. The flip side looks like this:

R - Receive

E - Every

S - Secret[291]

T - Treasure[292]

When you enter the secret place and *rest* in the safety of God's love, you honor God and your loss. Compassionately listening to your heart with the Holy Spirit, you find words and develop a language to communicate grief with emotional honesty.

As a truth-teller, you express what you believe, think, and feel about your loss, about God, yourself, and others. And you give yourself plenty of permission to release the unbearable pain into God's tender hands.

Emptied and surrendered to Love, little by little you gently release the various fragments of your pain. You listen, watch, and wait for your redeeming

Friend to grace you with higher-level perspective and timeless treasure.[293] So much more is happening *inside you* than the naked eye can see.

Following one of our traumatic losses, I discovered a slow, internal dismantling of how I defined myself, and my dreams attached to the future. I had no guarantee that the longings in my heart would ever be fulfilled.

I recall the words of my mentor, Dr. Pamela Reeve, who met with me once a month for many years until she passed away—still sharp as a tack, at ninety-five. In the comfort of her living room, she poured hot tea while I poured out the troubles of my heart. One afternoon, when shadows loomed especially dark, I shared something with her about the dismantling process I sensed happening inside me. She knew my story well.

Gently setting down her porcelain cup and saucer, she seemed to look straight through me. It was the same kind of look my grandmother used to give me—the one with the raised eyebrow that said, *Honey, I want you to pay very close attention.* With a tilt of her head she stated with the utmost confidence, "Pam, God never allows the breaking down of a vessel unless He intends to build it back up into something of greater value and capacity."

Instantly, I understood. She was challenging me to believe that the Holy Spirit was working deep inside me, beyond my puny discernment. She was encouraging me to rest in God's unconditional love and power to transform me from the inside out, in ways that exceeded my limited comprehension.[294]

I've never forgotten those words. And now, decades down the road, they ring truer than when I first heard them.

If you and I were to step together beyond time, pull back an imaginary curtain, and view your life today from eternity, we might see a tiny dot on a never-ending line. Let's say the small dot represents all the chapters of your life story, beginning to end. Certain sections detail your losses.

The view from this higher reference point allows you to see with greater clarity. With a full awareness of all the intricacies and minutiae encompassed in your story, God's intention has always been, and will always be, to replace your ashes with His beauty and bring life out of death.[295]

In the grip of grace, nothing is ever forced on you against your will. God invites you to participate *with* Him in redeeming loss, first your own, then in service to others.

Partnering with God through grief is a transformation experience, similar to a two-step or waltz. God leads, and you follow. The tempo, rhythm, and movements are choreographed uniquely for you, designed to ever-so-carefully orchestrate the way *through* your pain. Your Creator customizes your dance to connect, mend, liberate, revive and defy the tendency to hide in isolation.

As you dance, well-defined spiritual and mental shifts begin to appear *in* you. Moving in sync, hand in hand with Love, you're empowered to see with new eyes. Old preoccupations slowly fade away. Intuitive discernment grows, allowing you to notice nuances of God's goodness amidst the ordinary and mundane. Gratitude rises and joy pops up in a subtle new bounce in your step. Relationships progress, mature, and acquire new meaning.

Valuable treasures discovered in the dance empower you to flourish anew.

- The treasure of a *reset to linger and listen*. You make time to be still, to pay attention to your heart, and to give your feelings a voice. You turn toward your heartache with compassion, rather than denying, blocking, or running from it. Triggers and underlying needs are now an invitation to connect with yourself, with God and safe friends who may know you better than you know yourself. Being honest, open, and willing you engage in truth and love.

- The treasure of *Love Talks*. An inner knowing says, *this pain is bigger than me! I'm powerless to fix the devastation or to find my own way out of the blinding sadness.*

  In the safety of the secret place, the Holy Spirit gently nudges you out of the past and future, to bring you back to the present moment. You talk things over and sort things out with the One who loves you best and calls you friend.

  Legitimate grief is no longer an adversary you despise, fight, or shut out. It's a door of opportunity to learn, to grow, and to build intimacy with God who lives *in* you, eagerly waiting for you to reconnect. The terrain of loss is a place to mine gold by moonlight, discover priceless gems in timeless wisdom, and safely walk arm-in-arm with a guard and guide toward abundant wholeness.

- The treasure of *sharing your story*. You invite God and trusted friends into your story by sharing elements of your grief. You risk being vulnerable when it's safe, leaving behind the tendency to appear *fine* when you aren't. You let go of denying, pretending, avoiding, and hiding, in order to enjoy the benefits of living in the light: increased energy, improved health, emotional freedom, and deep, more fulfilling relationships.

- The treasure of *everlasting life*. Meaning is discovered in seeing your life in this world as a millisecond compared to the endless years of eternity. Between now and the time you leave here, you are being prepared for the realities of life everlasting.

  My mentor used to say, "God is using all the events from the smallest to the largest, from the happiest to the most horrific, to prepare you for your place in the new heaven and earth." This mystery boggles my mind. Obviously, my attempt to communicate the idea can't come close to conveying the power and brilliance of that future scene, when the old you seamlessly shifts into the new you, as Love carries you across the threshold to live happily, forever after.

Now, you may ask, can you unpack that for me? What in the world will that be like?

I must answer honestly: I haven't the foggiest. But if you like adventure you might hunt for clues in Scripture, read my friend Randy Alcorn's books, and let the Holy Spirit run with your imagination.

On the heels of loss, you may find yourself becoming more aware of the *opposites* that coexist in life. Experience tends to bring new meaning to the paradoxes we see around us.

Life in this world is bittersweet. Joy and sorrow are inseparable. Mystery lives in certainty.

Relief comes in being still. We slow our pace to accelerate our recovery.

We empty out to be filled afresh, releasing the old to receive the new.

First comes death, then resurrection. It's the message of the cross.

It's also the way of restoring and redeeming loss.

The point I'm moving toward is: *this is not the end of your story.* Your best chapters of flourishing and fulfillment are ahead. Creative renovations are happening deep *within you* that you have yet to realize or manifest. It's important to take good care of *you* and to trust God's goodness and timing in the process.

Partnering with God in healing your heart strategically sets the stage for your brighter future. Expect the process to be s-l-o-w and mercurial. Expect to shift from feeling better to exhausted to irritated and finicky in a wink. It goes with the territory. Don't let that throw you.

The mood swings will gradually narrow, soften, become less frequent, and eventually balance out. When you can't see a better future for yourself, let others carry your hope and envision it for you.

Through the years I've experienced excruciating grief, and yet, I've also tasted joyful pleasure in the simple things of life.

I've despised moments of feeling vulnerable and powerless; I much prefer feeling strong, capable, and in control. But I am learning— more slowly than I prefer —that control is really an illusion.

The bottom line? *It's not all up to us to make our lives work out.* Even the strange, the unplanned, and those things we call tragic can harmoniously weave together and bring forth beauty and goodness in the loving hands of God.

It's true. I've held private funerals to commemorate some of my own personal losses…

> *the death of agendas for my life and certain dreams I had for loved ones*
>
> *the death of a few professional positions*
>
> *the death of creative writing for years*
>
> *the death of once-cherished areas of influence*
>
> *the death of valued relationships and support, due to a lack of time, energy, and proximity*

Clearly, I have experienced times when my own soul felt dead.

But in the same breath, I can honestly say I have never felt more alive. New life is springing up through the sodden ashes of the old. I sense increased capacities and fresh vitality when I'm with family and friends or on assignment. New, previously undiscovered gifts have emerged that display ongoing evidence of mending miracles.

I am more at home with myself and others.

Faith, love, and acceptance have found deeper roots in my soul. I have increased confidence in God's goodness, and that *I am where I am supposed to be* at this time in my life. I rest in knowing that if God wants me in a different place, He'll strike up the music, invite me to waltz, and get me there right on time. So, I cling to this:

> *God is a redeeming genius who will dance you out of any pit into a life that flourishes with meaning and purpose.*[97]

I can't promise the dance will be fast, easy, effortless, or without risk. You are far too intricately created and valuable for false guarantees.

I can promise you a gentle dance that flows with mystery, grace-filled movement, powerful lifts and carries, and mesmerizing sails and catches that re-ignite passion and childlike wonder. These are the sacred ways of the Spirit who lives inside you, eager to love you back to life free and whole.[298]

It doesn't mean you don't feel sad now and then, or that you forget. It means you choose to live in the light and love in ways that honor God and your losses, because your precious life matters. There is only one *you* who can share your truth and fulfill the purposes designed by Love for your good and the good of others.

Joy in sorrow. Strength in weakness. Life in death.

Mending miracles. Heaven's glory streaming into torn, wounded, worn-out earthen vessels.[299]

It is God's signature on your life.

So, what will it be?

How will you respond when Love draws close and whispers: *Shall we dance?*

Endnote

Prologue

1. Hannah Donnelly is a talented singer songwriter, and daughter of my good friend, Jenny Donnelly. I've had the privilege to travel and speak with Jenny's Her Voice team across the United States.

2. Amy Grant was the first Contemporary Christian artist to have a platinum record, the first to hit No. 1 on the Pop charts and the first to perform at the GRAMMY® Awards. Her career spans more than 40 years and stretches from her roots in gospel into becoming an iconic singer, songwriter, television personality and philanthropist.

3. Job 33:14–15, NLT.

4. Cindy McGill is a creative rescue agent and world-wide influencer whose life and outreach stories never cease to leave me in awe of God. See her excellent book, Words that Work: *A Language of Light for a World Living in Darkness.*

5. I Cor 16:9, NLT. "There is a wide-open door for a great work here, although many oppose me."

6. Rev. 3:20, NLT. "Look! I stand at the door and knock. If you hear my voice and open the door, I will come in, and we will share a meal together as friends."

7   Col 4:3, GW. "Pray that God will give us an opportunity to speak the word so that we may tell the mystery about Christ."

8   Eph 5:1,2, NLT. Be imitators of God in everything you do, for then you will represent your Father as his beloved sons and daughters. And continue to walk surrendered to the extravagant love of Christ, for he surrendered his life as a sacrifice for us. His great love for us was pleasing to God, like an aroma of adoration—a sweet healing fragrance. *The Greek word imitate (*mimetes*) frequently depicts an actor playing a role. We are to mimic God, to see as he sees, think as he thinks, love as he loves, and act as he acts. (5:1). The Aramaic word for 'fragrance' can also be translated 'healing balm.' Fragrance – a combination of organic compounds that produce a distinctly sweet pleasant scent. A fragrance fills the senses and changes the atmosphere, activating parts of the brain that impact memory, mood, and emotion.

9   John 16:13, NIV. But when he, the Spirit of truth, comes, he will guide you into all the truth. He will not speak on his own; he will speak only what he hears, and he will tell you what is yet to come.

10   Gen 1:26, NLT. In the beginning Yahweh, the God of Israel, says, "Let us make humanity in our own image, in the likeness of ourselves" (Genesis 1:26). The use of the plural pronoun here reveals the nature of God as community. Father, Son, and Holy Spirit relate together in perfect harmony and unity. It is through our interactive relationship with God (giving and receiving) and within community, that we experience transformation and mind renewal. Peace and healing happen best in the context of healthy relationships (with God and others).

11   The Lord reminded me of these specific words spoken to me by Clyde Lewis during a prophetic prayer time with Jenny Donnelly.

12 Andy Crouch, *Strong and Weak: Embracing a Life of Love, Risk and True Flourishing* (Downers Grove, IL: InterVarsity Press, 2016), 40, 42. Andy is partner for theology and culture at Praxis, an organization that works as a creative engine for redemptive entrepreneurship. His work and writing have been featured in *The New York Times, The Wall Street Journal,* and *Time*.

Chapter 1

13 John 15:1-2, AMP

14 See this comprehensive resource by world leading expert on trauma, Bessel Van der Kolk, MD. *The Body Keeps Score: Brain, Mind, and Body in the Healing of Trauma,* (New York: Penguin Random House, 2015).

15 Benjamin P. Chapman et al., "Emotion suppression and mortality risk over a 12-year follow-up," *Journal of Psychosomatic Research* 75, no. 4 (2013): 381–85. https://doi.org/10.1016/j.jpsychores.2013.07.014.

16 J. Holt-Lunstad, T.B. Smith, and J.B. Layton, "Social Relationships and Mortality Risk: A Meta-analytic Review," *PLoS Med* 7, no. 7 (2010): e1000316. https://doi.org/10.1371/journal.pmed.1000316. An analysis of 148 research studies with more than 308,000 participants looked at how relationships impact health and mortality. The results showed that not having meaningful connections with family and friends can be as bad for a person's well-being as well-established risk factors such as smoking, alcoholism, physical inactivity, and obesity.

17 John Mark Comer, *Garden City: Work, Rest, and the Art of Being Human* (Nashville, TN: Thomas Nelson, 2017). This book is a must read by a brilliant young thought leader who lays out a Biblical view of 'calling' as the courage to do what God has created

us for, using the passions and skills he's given us, to make a unique impact in his world. John Mark Comer is a NY Times best-selling author of several books who offers a practical ground-breaking model and tools for spiritual transformation free of charge at practicingtheway.org. Discover treasure here!

18 Andy Crouch, *Strong and Weak: Embracing a Life of Love, Risk, and True Flourishing,* Intervarsity Press, p.10-11.

Chapter 2

19 M. C. Eisma et al., "Avoidance processes mediate the relationship between rumination and symptoms of complicated grief," *Journal of Abnormal Psychology* 122, no. 4 (2013): 961–70.

20 James W. Pennebaker, *Opening Up: The Healing Power of Expressing Emotions* (New York: Guilford Press, 1997), 2, 56.

21 Ibid., p.56.

22 Brain SPECT Imaging is a type of imaging test that uses nuclear medicine and a special camera to create 3D pictures of the brain's blood flow and activity.

23 Stephen Lepore and M. A. Greenberg, "Mending broken hearts," *Psychology and Health* 17 (2002): 547–60.

24 J. M. Smyth and M. A. Greenberg, "Scriptotherapy: the effects of writing about traumatic events," in *Empirical Studies in Psychoanalytic Theories,* vol. 9, eds. J. Maslig and P. Duberstien (Washington, DC: American Psychological Association, 2000), 121J.

25 J. W. Pennebaker, J. K. Kiecolt-Glaser and R. Glaser, "Disclosure of traumas and immune function. Health implications for psychotherapy," *Journal of Consulting and Clinical Psychology,* 56 (1988) pp. 239–245.

26. Lepore, Stephen J. Expressive writing moderates the relation between intrusive thoughts and depressive symptoms. *Journal of Personality and Social Psychology* 73, no. 5 (1997): 1030–37.

27. P. Ullrich and S. Lutgendorf, "Journaling about stressful events: Effects of cognitive processing and emotional expression," *Annals of Behavioral Medicine,* 24(3) (2002, February) pp. 244-250.

28. Pennebaker, James W., and Colder, Michelle and Sharp, Lisa K. *Accelerating the coping process. Journal of Personality and Social Psychology,* Vol 58(3), Mar 1990, 528-537.

29. Drake Baer, "Expressive writing is a super easy way to become way happier," *Business Insider* (May 23, 2014). Retrieved from www.businessinsider.com/the-positive-effects-of-journaling-and-expressive-writing-2014-5.

30. I Kings 19:11-13, NLT.

31. Maud Purcell, "The Health Benefits of Journaling," www.PsychCentral.com (October 30, 2015).

Chapter 3

32. Isaiah 42:3, NASB. The Message translation says this: He won't brush aside the bruised and the hurt and he won't disregard the small and insignificant, but he'll steadily and firmly set things right. He won't tire out and quit. He won't be stopped until he's finished his work—to set things right on earth.

33. Rachel Yehuda, PhD, professor of psychiatry, neuroscience, and director of traumatic stress studies at the Icahn School of Medicine at Mount Sinai, is a pioneer in understanding how the effects of stress and trauma can transmit biologically, beyond events, to the next generation.

34 Bessel van der Kolk, MD, is a leading expert in the treatment of trauma and how trauma affects the brain, body, and nervous system.

35 2 Cor 3:18, AMP. And we all, with unveiled face, *continually* seeing as in a mirror the glory of the Lord, are *progressively* being transformed into His image from [one degree of] glory to [even more] glory, which comes from the Lord, [who is] the Spirit.

36 Maud Purcell, "The Health Benefits of Journaling", www.PsychCentral.com (October 30, 2015).

37 P. A. Boelen, J. De Keijser, M. A. Van Den Hout and J. Van Den Bout, "Treatment of complicated grief: A comparison between cognitive-behavioral 234 therapy and supportive counseling," *Journal of Consulting and Clinical Psychology,* 75, (2007) pp. 277–284. doi: www.dx.doi.org/10.1037/0022-006X.75.2.277

38 N.M. Simon, "Treating complicated grief." *JAMA: The Journal of the American Medical Association.* 310 (2013):416–423. https://doi.org/10.1001/jama.2013.8614.

39 Psalm 23:6, NLT.

40 John Mark Comer, *Practicing the Way: Be with Jesus, Become like him, Do as he did.* (Waterbrook, 2024), p. 107.

41 Crouch, Andy. The Life We're Looking For: *Reclaiming Relationship in a Technological World.* 2022. Convergent, a division of Penguin Random House. On pages 33-35 Andy Crouch unpacks durable wisdom from the ancient Jewish Shema, extended by Jesus, and gives us a compact summary of what being fully human involves. Every person is a heart-soul-mind-strength complex designed for love. You are not a mind without a heart, or a brain without a body, or a body without a soul. You are all of these, together, and

it is this complex of qualities that makes you the unique person you are.

42 Contributed by Sarah Rodriguez, age 13, while healing after the loss of her father.

43 Contributed by Karen Bressel while partnering with God to conquer cancer.

44 Neimeyer, R.A., Burke, L.A., Mackay, M.M. and Van Dyke Stinger, J.G. (2010). Grief therapy and the reconstruction of meaning: From principles to practice. *Journal of Contemporary Psychotherapy,* 40(2), 73-83.

45 Y. A. Iliya, "Music Therapy as Grief Therapy for Adults with Mental Illness and Complicated Grief: A Pilot Study," *Death Studies* 39, no. 3 (2015): 173–184, https://doi.org/10.1080/07481187.2014.946623.

46 S. Porter, T. McConnell, M. Clarke, et al., "A Critical Realist Evaluation of a Music Therapy Intervention in Palliative Care," *BMC Palliative Care* 16 (2017): 70, https://doi.org/10.1186/s12904-017-025.

47 Tricia Fox Ransom, The Gathering (album), 2021, https://www.triciafoxmusic.com/the-gathering-album. See also: Tricia Fox Ransom, *Message in the Music: Do Lyrics Impact Well-Being?* Tricia's Capstone Thesis, 2021, has been downloaded over 100K times. As a singer-songwriter and thought leader on musical lyrics and well-being, Tricia facilitates song-writing sessions that foster self-worth and catharsis.

48 H. L. Stuckey and J. Nobel, "The Connection Between Art, Healing, and Public Health: A Review of Current Literature," *American Journal of Public Health* 100, no. 2 (2010): 254–263.

Chapter 4

49 National Academies of Sciences, Engineering, and Medicine. *Social Isolation and Loneliness in Older Adults: Opportunities for the Health Care System* (Washington, DC: The National Academies Press, 2020), https://doi.org/10.17226/25663.

50 Gen. 2:18, TLB. God said, "It's not good for the Man to be alone; I will make a companion for him, a helper suited to his needs."

51 "Social Isolation and Loneliness in Older Adults," *American Journal of Epidemiology* 188, no. 1 (January 2019): 102–109, https://doi.org/10.1093/aje/kwy231.

52 National Academies of Sciences, Engineering, and Medicine. 2020. *Social Isolation and Loneliness in Older Adults: Opportunities for the Health Care System.* Washington, DC: The National Academies Press. https://doi.org/10.17226/25663.

53 Tish Harrison Warren, *Prayer in the Night: For Those Who Work or Watch or Weep* (IL: InterVarsity Press, 2021), 19.

54 Psalm 34:18, NLT. The Lord is close to the brokenhearted; he rescues those whose spirits are crushed.

55 I Peter 1:17, NLT. And remember that the heavenly Father to whom you pray has no favorites.

56 2 Cor 12:9-10, AMP. He has said to me, "My grace is sufficient for you [My lovingkindness and My mercy are more than enough—always available—regardless of the situation]; for [My] power is being perfected [and is completed and shows itself most effectively] in [your] weakness." Therefore, I will all the more gladly boast in my weaknesses, so that the power of Christ [may completely enfold me and] may dwell in me. 10 So I am well pleased with weaknesses, with insults, with distresses, with persecutions, and

with difficulties, for the sake of Christ; for when I am weak [in human strength], then I am strong [truly able, truly powerful, truly drawing from God's strength].

57 Dallas Willard, The *Divine Conspiracy: Rediscovering Our Hidden Life in God* (San Francisco: Harper, 1998); and *The Spirit of the Disciplines: Understanding How God Changes Lives* (San Francisco: Harper, 1988). For a more comprehensive overview of what life is meant to be with Jesus in the kingdom of God, see these classics by Dallas Willard. Dallas was a brilliant thought leader attuned to the heart of God and popular professor who taught at the University of Southern California nearly 50 years.

58 Matt. 11:28-30, MSG. Is 55:3, NLT, Come to me with your ears wide open. Listen, and you will find life.

59 I'm grateful to Clyde Lewis, Professional Coach and Chaplain for the Portland, Oregon Police Bureau, for encouraging me to ask these questions, especially when my inner world is messy and difficult to understand.

60 My thanks to Richard Rhorer for offering this challenge during his keynote address at the American Association of Christian Counselors World Conference, Nashville, Tennessee. It's a profound insight I've never forgotten.

61 Zeph. 3:17, TLB. For the Lord your God has arrived to live among you. He is a mighty Savior. He will give you victory. He will rejoice over you with great gladness; he will love you and not accuse you. Is that a joyous choir I hear? No, it is the Lord himself exulting over you in happy song. 'I have gathered your wounded and taken away your reproach.'; Matt. 28:20, NLT, And be sure of this: I am with you always, even to the end of the age.

62 Psalm 34:18, NLT. The Lord is close to the brokenhearted; he rescues those whose spirits are crushed.

63 John 15:15, MSB. Jesus said, I do not communicate with you on a slave – boss basis; slaves have no clue what their Master is about to do. I talk to you as my friends telling you everything that I have heard in my conversation and intimate association with my Father. This I explain to you in the clearest possible terms.

Chapter 5

64 Genesis 1:2, ESV. The earth was without form and void, and darkness was over the face of the deep. And the Spirit of God was hovering over the face of the waters.

65 Gen 2:7, ESV

66 Job 33:4, ESV.

67 Yilmaz Balban, M., Cafaro, E., Saue-Fletcher, L., Washington, M. J., Bijanzadeh, M., Lee, A. M., Chang, E. F., and Huberman, A. D. "Human Responses to Visually Evoked Threat." *Current Biology* 31 (2021): 601–612.e3. https://doi.org/10.1016/j.cub.2020.11.035.

68 "Fight, flight, or freeze" is an automatic physiological reaction that occurs in response to a perceived threat or danger and is often referenced in trauma and psychology literature. *Fight* is the body's way of facing a threat aggressively, such as by physically fighting or verbally saying "No." *Flight* is the body's way of moving away from danger, such as by running, hiding, or backing away. *Freeze* is the body's way of becoming immobile and unable to act against a threat, such as by going tense, still, and silent.

69 Perl, O., Ravia, A., Rubinson, M., Eisen, A., Soroka, T., Mor, N., Secundo, L., and Sobel, N. "Human Non-Olfactory Cognition

Phase-Locked with Inhalation." *Nature Human Behaviour* 3 (2019): 501–512. https://doi.org/10.1038/s41562-019-0556-z.

70 Herbert Benson, *The Relaxation Response* (New York: William Morrow & Co., 1975). For a deep dive into the science see Dr. Herbert Benson's research here. In the laboratories of Harvard Medical School, Dr. Benson and colleagues discovered this revitalizing, therapeutic technique, now routinely recommended to treat patients suffering from stress and anxiety, including heart conditions, high blood pressure, chronic pain, insomnia, and many other physical and psychological ailments. Dr. Benson, a renowned Cardiologist, introduced this approach to relieving stress over forty years ago.

71 Ma, Xiao, Yue Zi-Qi, Gong Zhu-Qing, Zhang Hong, Duan Nai-Yue, Shi Yu-Tong, Wei Gao-Xia, and Li You-Fa. "The Effect of Diaphragmatic Breathing on Attention, Negative Affect and Stress in Healthy Adults." *Frontiers in Psychology* 8 (2017). https://doi.org/10.3389/fpsyg.2017.00874.

72 Chen, Y.-F., Huang, X.-Y., Chien, C.-H., and Cheng, J.-F. "The Effectiveness of Diaphragmatic Breathing Relaxation Training for Reducing Anxiety." *Perspectives in Psychiatric Care* 53 (2017): 329–336. https://doi.org/10.1111/ppc.12184.

73 Stephen Porges. "The Polyvagal Theory: New Insights into Adaptive Reactions of the Autonomic Nervous System." *Cleveland Clinic Journal of Medicine* 76, Suppl. 2 (April 2009).

74 Psalm 46:10, NLT. Be still, and know that I am God!

75 Caroline Sevoz-Couche and Sylvian Laborde. "Heart Rate Variability and Slow-Paced Breathing: When Coherence Meets Resonance." *Neuroscience & Biobehavioral Reviews* 135 (2022). https://doi.org/10.1016/j.neubiorev.2022.104576.

76. Box Breathing: Inhale for a count of four, hold for four, exhale for four, hold for four. Easy to use anytime, anywhere.

77. Tactical Breathing: Inhale to a count of four, pause briefly, and exhale to a count of eight. Repeat several times

78. Cyclic Sighing: Inhale through the nose fully, then inhale again briefly before a long, full exhale by mouth; repeat for 5 minutes.

79. Melis Yilmaz Balban et al. "Brief Structured Respiration Practices Enhance Mood and Reduce Physiological Arousal." *Cell Reports Medicine* (January 17, 2023).

80. For additional science-based breathing practices go to https://pamvredevelt.com/breathwork

81. Christina Zelano et al. "Nasal Respiration Entrains Human Limbic Oscillations and Modulates Cognitive Function." *Journal of Neuroscience* 36, no. 49 (December 7, 2016): 12448–12467. https://doi.org/10.1523/JNEUROSCI.2586-16.2016.

82. Hong Y. G., Kim H. K., Son Y. D., and Kang C. K. "Identification of Breathing Patterns through EEG Signal Analysis Using Machine Learning." *Brain Sciences* 11, no. 3 (February 26, 2021): 293. https://doi.org/10.3390/brainsci11030293.

83. Carol Williams, "How to Breathe Your Way to Better Memory and Sleep," *New Scientist*, January 8, 2020.

84. James Nestor, *Breath: The New Science of a Lost Art* (New York: Riverhead Books, 2020). For a comprehensive review of the history and science on why and how breathing determines our life capacity see this book by James Nestor.

85　Jer. 6:16, NIV. This is what the Lord says: "Stand at the crossroads and look; ask for the ancient paths, ask where the good way is, and walk in it, and you will find rest for your souls."

86　I Thes. 5:17, ESV

87　See Luke 18:10-14 and Mark 10:46-52

88　Refer to Psalm 118:1. Inhale with "Give thanks to the Lord; Exhale with "His love endures forever."

89　Rev. John Breck, "From the Prayer of Jesus to Prayer of the Heart," *Orthodox Church in America* Newsletter, May 11, 2010. https://www.oca.org/reflections/fr.-john-breck/from-the-prayer-of-jesus-to-prayer-of-the-heart. Fr. Breck was Professor of New Testament and Ethics at St. Vladimir's Seminary and Professor of Biblical Interpretation and Ethics at St. Sergius Theological Institute, Paris, France. With his wife, Lyn, he is the director of the St. Silouan Retreat Center, Wadmalaw Island, South Carolina.

Chapter 6

90　John Mark Comer, *Practicing the Way: Be with Jesus, Become Like Him, Do as He Did* (Colorado Springs, CO: Waterbrook, 2024), 103. For free companion videos and excellent training materials, see https://www.practicingtheway.org.

91　John 8:32, NLT

Chapter 7

92　John 9:1-3, MSG.

93　Jeremiah 29:11-13, NLT.

94. Eph. 2:10, NLT. For we are God's masterpiece. He has created us anew in Christ Jesus, so we can do the good things he planned for us long ago.

Chapter 8

95. Psalm 31:15, NIV. My times are in your hands.

96. Philippians 4:11-13, MSG. I've *learned* by now to be quite content whatever my circumstances. I'm just as happy with little as with much, with much as with little. I've found the recipe for being happy whether full or hungry, hands full or hands empty. Whatever I have, wherever I am, I can make it through anything in the One who makes me who I am.

97. Kristin Neff, "Tips for Practicing Self-Compassion," accessed June 2024, https://self-compassion.org/tips-for-practice/.

98. Rick Hanson, *Hardwiring Happiness: The New Brain Science of Contentment, Calm, and Confidence* (New York: Harmony Books, 2013). Dr. Hanson is a neuropsychologist. In this book he describes the process by which the brain can be reshaped (positive neuroplasticity) and highlights the idea that what you pay attention to, and rest your mind on, is the primary shaper of your brain. It correlates with timeless wisdom that directs us to set our minds on God. Is. 26:3, ESV. You keep him in perfect peace whose mind is stayed on you, because he trusts in you.

99. Pete Scazzero, "Know Yourself that You May Know God," Part 2, *Emotionally Healthy Spirituality Course* (2015), 2. https://www.emotionallyhealthy.org/wp-content/uploads/2015/10/Session-2-Know-Yourself-Know-God.pdf

100. Matthew Tull and Nathan Kimbrel, "Emotion in Posttraumatic Stress Disorder: Etiology, Assessment, Neurobiology, and

101 Psalm 34:18, ESV. The Lord is near to the brokenhearted and saves the crushed in spirit.

102 2 Cor. 12:10, J.B. PHILLIPS. The Lord's reply has been, "My grace is enough for you: for where there is weakness, my power is shown the more completely." Therefore, I have cheerfully made up my mind to be proud of my weaknesses, because they mean a deeper experience of the power of Christ. I can even enjoy weaknesses, suffering, privations, persecutions and difficulties for Christ's sake. For my very weakness makes me strong in him.

103 Psalm 145:19, TLB. He fulfills the desires of those who reverence and trust him; he hears their cries for help and rescues them.

104 Exodus 34:6, NIV.

105 A. W. Tozer, *The Knowledge of the Holy* (New York: HarperCollins, 1961), 91.

106 Luke 7:11-17, NLT.

107 Acts 10:38, NLT.

108 Luke 4:18, NLT.

109 The word *compassion* is used seven times in the Gospels in reference to Jesus's emotions as compared to sorrow, anger, and gratitude mentioned four times, love stated three times, and joy used twice.

110 John 11:32-34, AMP. When Mary came to the place where Jesus was and saw Him, she fell at His feet, saying to Him, "Lord, if You had been here, my brother would not have died." When Jesus saw

her sobbing, and the Jews who had come with her also sobbing, He was *deeply moved* in spirit to the point of anger at the sorrow caused by death and was troubled, and said, "Where have you laid him?" They said, "Lord, come and see." * (The term *deeply moved* suggests an emotional indignation or sternness. Jesus was angry at the sorrow caused by death. It occurs four more times in the NT in reference to Jesus' words or His feelings. See Matt 9:30; Mark 1:43; John 11:38; 13:21)

111 Ephesians 3:16,17, NLT. I pray that from his glorious, unlimited resources he will empower you with inner strength through his Spirit. Then Christ will make his home in your hearts as you trust in him. Your roots will grow down into God's love and keep you strong. And may you have the power to understand, as all God's people should, how wide, how long, how high, and how deep his love is.

112 Teresa of Avila, *The Interior Castle*, 1:2.8, in *Collected Works*, vol. 2, trans. Kieran Kavanaugh and Otillo Rodriguez (Washington, DC: ICS Publications, 1980), 291.

113 John O'Donohue, "The Presence of Compassion," interview by Mary NurrieStearns, *Personal Transformation*, accessed Feb. 2024, https://www.personaltransformation.com/johnodonohue.html. John O'Donohue was an Irish poet, author, and Priest. At the heart of John's awakened beliefs was the premise that ancient wisdom could offer desperately needed nourishment for the spiritual hunger experienced in our modern world.

114 I John 3:18-24, The MSG. My dear children, let's not just talk about love; let's practice real love. This is the only way we'll know we're living truly, living in God's reality. It's also the way to shut down debilitating self-criticism, even when there is something to it. For God is greater than our worried hearts and knows more

about us than we do ourselves. And friends, once that's taken care of and we're no longer accusing or condemning ourselves, we're bold and free before God! We're able to stretch our hands out and receive what we asked for because we're doing what he said, doing what pleases him. Again, this is God's command: to believe in his personally named Son, Jesus Christ. He told us to love each other, in line with the original command. As we keep his commands, we live deeply and surely in him, and he lives in us. And this is how we experience his deep and abiding presence in us: by the Spirit he gave us.

115 Elaine Beaumont, Adam Galpin, and Peter Jenkins, "Being Kinder to Myself: A Prospective Comparative Study, Exploring Post-Trauma Therapy Outcome Measures," *Counselling Psychology Review* 27, no. 1 (2012).

116 Nef, Kristin (2003) *Self-Compassion: An Alternative Conceptualization of a Healthy Attitude Toward Oneself*, Psychology Press, Self and Identity, 2: 85–101.

117 Angus MacBeth and Andrew Gumley, "Exploring Compassion: A Meta-Analysis of the Association Between Self-Compassion and Psychopathology," *Clinical Psychology Review* 32, no. 6 (2012): 545–552.

118 M. Khursheed and M. G. Shahnawaz, "Trauma and Post-Traumatic Growth: Spirituality and Self-Compassion as Mediators Among Parents Who Lost Their Young Children in a Protracted Conflict," *Journal of Religion and Health* 59 (2020): 2623–2637.

119 Augustine, *Confessions*. Augustine believed that knowledge of God and knowledge of oneself are deeply intertwined. He was persuaded that true self-knowledge is an essential step in drawing closer to God and growing closer to God empowers greater self-knowledge.

120 Kristin Neff, "Self-Compassion: An Alternative Conceptualization of a Healthy Attitude Toward Oneself," *Self and Identity* 2, no. 2 (2003): 85–101.

121 Isaiah 42:16, AMP. I will lead the blind by a way they do not know; I will guide them in paths that they do not know. I will make darkness into light before them and rugged places into plains. These things I will do [for them], and I will not leave them abandoned *or* undone.

122 Col. 3:13, NIV. Bear with each other and forgive one another if any of you has a grievance against someone (*this includes yourself*). Forgive as the Lord forgave you.

123 Proverbs 4:23, NLT. Guard your heart above all else, for it determines the course of your life.

124 Proverbs 3:5-8, MSG. Trust God from the bottom of your heart; don't try to figure out everything on your own. Listen for God's voice in everything you do, everywhere you go; he's the one who will keep you on track. Don't assume that you know it all. Run to God! Run from evil! Your body will glow with health; your very bones will vibrate with life!

125 2 Cor 3:17-18, ESV. Now the Lord is the Spirit, and where the Spirit of the Lord is, there is freedom. And we all, with unveiled face, reflecting the glory of the Lord, are being transformed into the same image from one degree of glory to another. For this comes from the Lord who is the Spirit.

126 I Cor. 1:8-9, NLT. He will keep you strong to the end so that you will be free from all blame… God will do this, for he is faithful to do what he says, and he has invited you into partnership with his Son, Jesus Christ our Lord.

127   Eph. 3:20, NLT. Now all glory to God, who is able, through his mighty power at work within us, to accomplish infinitely more than we might ask or think.

Chapter 10

128   Psalm 91:11-12, TLB. For he orders his angels to protect you wherever you go. They will steady you with their hands to keep you from stumbling against the rocks on the trail.

Chapter 11

129   Years later, I came across details that catalyzed a fresh sense of wonder related to this part of our story. Connections I hadn't noticed before, tied to the specific timing of our encounters, suddenly stood out like pieces of a divine puzzle. It was as if God had been gently threading golden strands of meaning through moments I didn't fully understand. Looking back, I now see His fingerprints more clearly, and it has deepened my sense of trust. The insights from two Scriptures and rabbinical teachings on the symbolic meaning of numbers are listed for you here.:

1. Matthew 14:24-25, NLT. "Meanwhile, the disciples were in trouble far away from land, for a strong wind had risen, and they were fighting heavy waves. About *three o'clock in the morning* Jesus came toward them, walking on the water."

2. Matthew 27:45-46, NLT. "At noon, darkness fell across the whole land until *three o'clock*. At about *three o'clock*, Jesus called out with a loud voice, "Eli, Eli lema sabachthani?" which means "My God, my God, why have you abandoned me?"

3. In Rabbinical teachings, the number three symbolizes completeness, wholeness, resurrection, and harmony in the Bible. It also represents the Holy Trinity, and is often associated with

divine importance. The number three is repeated over 450 times in Scripture and is used in the Torah to mediate between two opposing or contradictory values. The third value mediates, reconciles, and synthesizes the two into perfect union. Three is the number of truth and connection. *https://www.betemunah.org/three.html

130 Col. 2:2-3, GNT. I do this in order that they may be filled with courage and may be drawn together in love, and so have the full wealth of assurance which true understanding brings. In this way they will know God's secret, which is Christ himself. He is the key that opens all the hidden treasures of God's wisdom and knowledge.

131 I Cor 12:4-7, MSG. God's various gifts are handed out everywhere; but they all originate in God's Spirit. God's various ministries are carried out everywhere; but they all originate in God's Spirit. God's various expressions of power are in action everywhere; but God himself is behind it all. Each person is given something to do that shows who God is: Everyone gets in on it, everyone benefits.

132 Diane Russell, oil painting commissioned by the author, based on Jessie's vision of Nathan and Jesus. Adapted by request to depict a natural setting. Diane Russell is an award-winning portrait artist based in Portland, Oregon. Her work can be viewed at https://www.dianerussell.net or by contacting diane@dianerussell.net.

Chapter 12

133 Deuteronomy 2:7, NASB

134 Psalm 56:8, MSG

135 Psalm 56:11-13, MSG

136 Luke 15:11-32, MSG

Chapter 13

137 I Cor. 2:9-10, NLT. That is what the Scriptures mean when they say, "No eye has seen, no ear has heard, and no mind has imagined what God has prepared for those who love him." But it was to us that God revealed these things by his Spirit. For his Spirit searches out everything and shows us God's deep secrets. When we tell you these things, we do not use words that come from human wisdom. Instead, we speak words given to us by the Spirit, using the Spirit's words to explain spiritual truths.

138 John 14:22-23, AMP. Lord, how is it that You will reveal Yourself [make Yourself real] to us and not to the world? Jesus answered, If a person [really] loves Me, he will keep My word [obey My teaching]; and My Father will love him, and We will come to him and make Our home (abode, special dwelling place) with him.

139 Isaiah 58:9, 11, AMP. Then you will call, and the Lord will answer; You will cry for help, and He will say, "Here I am"... And the Lord will continually guide you, and satisfy your soul in scorched *and* dry places, And give strength to your bones; And you will be like a watered garden, And like a spring of water whose waters do not fail.

140 I John 2:20, AMP. But you have an anointing from the Holy One [you have been set apart, specially gifted and prepared by the Holy Spirit], and all of you know [the truth because He teaches us, illuminates our minds, and guards us from error].

141 Matt 6:22, AMP. The eye is the lamp of the body; so, if your eye is clear [spiritually perceptive], your whole body will be full of light [benefiting from God's precepts].

142 Gal. 5:22-23, MSG. But what happens when we live God's way? He brings gifts into our lives, much the same way that fruit appears in an orchard—things like affection for others, exuberance

about life, serenity. We develop a willingness to stick with things, a sense of compassion in the heart, and a conviction that a basic holiness permeates things and people. We find ourselves involved in loyal commitments, not needing to force our way in life, able to marshal and direct our energies wisely.

143. Rev. 3:20, TLB. Look! I have been standing at the door, and I am constantly knocking. If anyone hears me calling him and opens the door, I will come in and fellowship with him and he with me.

144. Phil. 4:6,7, AMP. Do not be anxious or worried about anything, but in everything [every circumstance and situation] by prayer and petition with thanksgiving, continue to make your [specific] requests known to God. 7 And the peace of God [that peace which reassures the heart, that peace] which transcends all understanding, [that peace which] stands guard over your hearts and your minds in Christ Jesus [is yours].

Chapter 14

145. I Sam. 16:13, NLT. So as David stood there among his brothers, Samuel took the flask of olive oil he had brought and anointed David with the oil. And the Spirit of the Lord came powerfully upon David from that day on.

146. I Sam. 13:14 AMP. The Lord has sought out for Himself a man (David) after His own heart, and the Lord has appointed him as leader *and* ruler over His people, because you have not kept (obeyed) what the Lord commanded you. Acts 1:22, NLT. But God removed Saul and replaced him with David, a man about whom God said, 'I have found David, son of Jesse, a man after my own heart. He will do everything I want him to do.'

147 Victor H. Matthews and Dan Pioske, "David," *Oxford Bibliographies*, last modified May 26, 2023, https://doi.org/10.1093/OBO/9780195393361-0027.

148 Psalm 42:6, VOICE. My God, my soul is so traumatized; the only help is remembering You wherever I may be.

149 Psalm 56:8, TLB. You have seen me tossing and turning through the night. You have collected all my tears and preserved them in your bottle! You have recorded each one in your book.

150 Psalm 27:4, AMP Classic

151 Psalm 27:8, NLT

152 For a clear picture of how David's conversations with God affected his choices and outcomes read I Samuel 23, 2 Samuel 5:19-25, 2 Sam. 30:8-18. Notice the questions David asks God, and how God answered specifically.

153 Jamie Winship, *Living Fearlessly: Exchanging the Lies of the World for the Liberating Truths of God* (Grand Rapids, MI: Revell, 2022), 79–81. For more about Jamie and Donna Winship's exceptional training and consulting work, visit https://www.identityexchange.com. These esteemed global thought leaders inspire individuals and teams to unlock deeper creativity and resilience, all within the empowering framework of true identity.

154 See the story at the beginning of I Sam. 23, NLT.

155 I Sam. 27:1, NLT. But *David kept thinking to himself,* "Someday Saul is going to get me. The best thing I can do is escape to the Philistines." David is worn out. He has been on the run under intense pressure for years. It seemed like he was nearing his end and that he'd never survive Saul's threats. In his wearied state of mind, he sees his death as the only option. Rather than pausing to talk

things over with God, David kept thinking to himself, and makes a rash decision that escorts him, his family and fellow soldiers into greater troubles. Shortly before this David was confident that God protected his life (I Sam. 24:15). Abigail assured him this was true (I Sam. 25:29). But now David speaks of death as a pending reality if he does not flee to the land of the Philistines, which is Israel's archenemy (27:1). David had previously declared that Saul would perish (26:10). After *thinking to himself* he says that *he is the one* who will perish. Though David begged the king not to force him from his home country, now he is compelled to run even though Saul has given him some assurance of safety.

156 Bob Deffinbaugh, *A Study of I Samuel: One Step Forward and Two Backward (1 Samuel 27:1–28:2) or What's a Man Like You Doing in a Place Like This?*, Bible.org, accessed July 2023, https://bible.org/seriespage/one-step-forward-and-two-backward-1-samuel-271-282-or-what-s-man-you-doing-place.

157 David's community supported and helped David sustain this habit. Part of his kingly routine was to hand copy the Torah, the first five books of the Bible, in company with a priest, and to read it daily. The process is described in Deut.17:18-20, TLB. And when he has been crowned and sits upon his throne as king, then he must copy these laws from the book kept by the Levite-priests. That copy of the laws shall be his constant companion. He must read from it every day of his life so that he will learn to respect the Lord his God by obeying all of his commands. This regular reading of God's laws will prevent him from feeling that he is better than his fellow citizens. It will also prevent him from turning away from God's laws in the slightest respect and will ensure his having a long, good reign. His sons will then follow him upon the throne.

158   Psalm 51:1. VOICE. Look on me with a heart of mercy, O God, according to Your generous love. According to Your great compassion, wipe out *every consequence of* my *shameful crimes*.

159   Psalm 38:5,6,8,15, ESV. My wounds stink and fester because of my foolishness, I am utterly bowed down and prostrate; all the day I go about mourning. I am feeble and crushed; I groan because of the tumult of my heart. But for you, O Lord, do I wait; it is you, O Lord my God, who will answer.

160   Psalm 91:1-2, NKJV.

161   Technostress is typically driven by five factors: techno-overload, techno-invasion, techno-complexity, techno-insecurity and techno-incertitude. Techno-overload refers to the need to process information of multiple tasks simultaneously using technological devices. Techno-invasion occurs when technology invades personal life and privacy, generating the constant need to be connected anywhere and at all times. Techno-complexity is defined as the complexity associated with the use of information computer technology (ICT), which implies spending time and effort to learn how to use them effectively. Techno-insecurity is the feeling that technology threatens job stability and maintenance of employment. Techno-incertitude comes from the constant updates and changes in ICT.

162   U.S. Department of Health and Human Services, Office of the U.S. Surgeon General. *Social Media and Youth Mental Health: The U.S. Surgeon General's Advisory* (2023), 5–8. https://www.hhs.gov/sites/default/files/sg-youth-mental-health-social-media-advisory.pdf.

163   Ibid.

164. Sharon Horwood and Jeromy Anglim, "Problematic Smartphone Usage and Subjective and Psychological Well-Being," *Computers in Human Behavior* 97 (2019): 44–50.

165. Psalm 139:1-6, NASB. Lord, You have searched me and known *me*. You know when I sit down and when I get up; You understand my thought from far away. You scrutinize my path and my lying down, and are acquainted with all my ways. Even before there is a word on my tongue, behold, Lord, You know it all. You have encircled me behind and in front, and placed Your hand upon me. *Such* knowledge is too wonderful for me; it is *too* high, I cannot comprehend it.

166. Psalm 139:23-24, TLB. Search me, O God, and know my heart; test my thoughts. Point out anything you find in me that makes you sad, and lead me along the path of everlasting life.

167. I Peter 4:8, ESV. Above all, keep loving one another earnestly, since love covers a multitude of sins.

168. See Psalm 32

169. Psalm 91:1,2, NKJV. He who dwells in the secret place of the Most High shall abide under the shadow of the Almighty. I will say of the Lord, "*He is* my refuge and my fortress; My God, in Him I will trust."

170. Isaiah 9:6, NLT. For a child is born to us, a son is given to us. The government will rest on his shoulders. And he will be called: Wonderful Counselor, Mighty God, Everlasting Father, Prince of Peace.

171. Psalm 34:18, NLT. The Lord is close to the brokenhearted; he rescues those whose spirits are crushed. *Jehovah-Rapha* has the power to heal physically (Psalm 41:3), emotionally (Psalm 147:3), mentally (Daniel 4:34), and spiritually (Psalm 103:2-3). *Rapha* in

Hebrew means not only 'healer,' but also 'to mend, cure, repair thoroughly, make whole.'

172 Luke 8:18, NLT. So pay attention to how you hear. To those who listen to my teaching, more understanding will be given.

173 Eph. 3:16-19, NLT. I pray that from his glorious, unlimited resources he will empower you with inner strength through his Spirit. 17 Then Christ will make his home in your hearts as you trust in him. Your roots will grow down into God's love and keep you strong. 18 And may you have the power to understand, as all God's people should, how wide, how long, how high, and how deep his love is. 19 May you experience the love of Christ, though it is too great to understand fully. Then you will be made complete with all the fullness of life and power that comes from God.

174 James 1:5, Voice. If you don't have all the wisdom needed for this journey, then all you have to do is ask God for it; and God will grant all that you need. He gives lavishly and never scolds you for asking.

175 James 3:17, NLT. But the wisdom from above is first of all pure. It is also peace loving, gentle at all times, and willing to yield to others. It is full of mercy and the fruit of good deeds. It shows no favoritism and is always sincere.

176 John 10:25, NLT. My sheep listen to my voice; I know them, and they follow me.

177 A. W. Tozer, *The Pursuit of God* (Camp Hill, PA: Christian Publications, 1993), 49.

178 Psalm 40:6, MSG. You've opened my ears so I can listen.

179 Isaiah 48:12-13, TLB. Listen to me, my people, my chosen ones! I alone am God. I am the First; I am the Last. It was my hand

that laid the foundations of the earth; the palm of my right hand spread out the heavens above; I spoke and they came into being. Come, all of you, and listen.

180 Dallas Willard, *Hearing God: Developing a Conversational Relationship with God* (Downers Grove, IL: InterVarsity Press, 1999), 9.

181 Frank Laubach and Brother Lawrence, *Practicing His Presence*, Library of Spiritual Classics, Vol. 1, ed. Gene Edwards (Georgia: The Seed Sowers, 1973), 46.

182 C. S. Lewis, *Mere Christianity* (New York: Macmillan, 1978), 167.

183 Romans 12:1,2. MSG. So here's what I want you to do, God helping you: Take your everyday, ordinary life—your sleeping, eating, going-to-work, and walking-around life—and place it before God as an offering. Embracing what God does for you is the best thing you can do for him. Don't become so well-adjusted to your culture that you fit into it without even thinking. Instead, fix your attention on God. You'll be changed from the inside out. Readily recognize what he wants from you, and quickly respond to it. Unlike the culture around you, always dragging you down to its level of immaturity, God brings the best out of you, develops well-formed maturity in you.

184 John 16:13-15, Voice. The Spirit of truth will come and guide you in all truth. He will not speak His own words to you; He will speak what He hears, revealing to you the things to come and bringing glory to Me. The Spirit has unlimited access to Me, to all that I possess and know, just as everything the Father has is Mine. That is the reason I am confident He will care for My own and reveal the path to you.

185 Isaiah 26:3, AMPC. You will guard him *and* keep him in perfect and constant peace whose mind [both its inclination and its character] is stayed on You, because he commits himself to You, leans on You, *and* hopes confidently in You.

186 Isaiah 1:18, NASB.

187 C. S. Lewis, *Miracles* (New York: Harper One, 2001), 65.

188 *Ibid.*, 65.

189 Tolkien, J. R., Unidentified attribution.

190 Isaiah 53:17. NIV

191 Eph. 1:18-20, GNT. I ask that your minds may be opened to see his light, so that you will know what is the hope to which he has called you, how rich are the wonderful blessings he promises his people, 19 and how very great is his power at work in us who believe. This power working in us is the same as the mighty strength 20 which he used when he raised Christ from death and seated him at his right side in the heavenly world.

192 Psalm 34:18, Voice. When someone is hurting or brokenhearted, the Eternal moves in close and revives him in his pain.

193 Luke 11:9-13, MSB. So what I'm saying to you is this, in prayer, it is the same, simple principle! Ask and it shall be given you; seek and you shall find; knock and it shall be opened for you. This is not just true for you as my friends [like in the parable], it is true even for those who are still total strangers to the Father's goodness! Everyone who asks will receive, and whoever searches will find and whoever knocks, the door will be opened! So, if you, even within the confines of an earth-bound, performance-based religious society, know to give your children excellent gifts that will only advantage them, how much more certainly will your

Father give the Holy Spirit out of his limitless, heavenly resources to everyone who asks him! ([1] The word, ὑπάρχω 1huparchō below rule - suggests the earth-dimension. [2] Again, the word often translated, evil, 2ponēros, means full of hardships and labors and annoyances which describes the typical performance-based religious society.)

194 James 1:17, MSB. Without exception God's 1gifts are only good; its perfection cannot be flawed. They come from 2above [where we originate from]; proceeding like light rays from its source, the Father of lights, with whom there is no distortion, or even a shadow of shifting to obstruct, or intercept the light; nor any hint of a hidden agenda. ([1] The principle of a 1gift, puts reward-language out of business. [2] The word, 2anouthen, means, from above. John 3:3, 13.)

195 John 14:23, NLT. Jesus answered him, This is so much more than a mere casual, distant and suspicious, or indifferent observation of me; this is about someone's 1passionate, loving desire, finding its rest in me; they will treasure my words and encounter my Father's love reflecting in them, and my Father and I will 2appear 3face to face to them, and make our 4abode 5with them. ([1] To love passionately, αγαπαω 1agapaō from agō and paō, to lead to rest [Psalm 23 in one word] - this word also links to the Hebrew word for love, בהא Ahab, to love with passionate desire; like a beating heart or breathing chest. Genesis 22;2 Abraham's love for Isaac. Jeremiah 31:3 I have loved you with an everlasting love: therefore with lovingkindness have I drawn you; [2] And we will appear [ἔρχομαι 2erchomai] face to face [pros] to this one; [3] The preposition, 3pros, as in John 1:1, face to face; [4] My Father and I will make our abode, 4monē, the same Greek word that is rendered mansions in the KJV in the verse 2 of this chapter. It is used nowhere else. The verb form, menō suggests a

seamless union. [John uses menō more than anyone else.] As in the next chapter, John 15:4. ...the branch abiding in the vine. God doesn't dwell in buildings made by human hands - God has no other address but 'you'-man life; [5] The word 5para expresses the closest possible nearness; a thing proceeding from a sphere of influence, with a suggestion of union of place of residence, to have sprung from its author and giver, originating from, denoting the point from which an action originates, intimate connection. The same constant that is enjoyed in the fellowship of the Father and the Son is yours. Jesus replied, All who love me will do what I say. My Father will love them, and we will come and make our home with each of them.

196 Laubach, Frank, and Brother Lawrence. *Practicing His Presence.* Library of Spiritual Classics, Vol. 1. Georgia: The Seed Sowers, 1973, 22.

Chapter 15

197 Lewis, C. S. *A Grief Observed.* New York: Harper One, 2015, 9-10.

198 John 10:10, ESV. The thief comes only to steal and kill and destroy. I came that they may have life and have it abundantly.

199 Warren, Tish Harrison, 2021. *Prayer in the Night for Those Who Work or Watch or Weep.* InterVasity Press, Downers Grove, Illinois, p.161.

200 2 Kings 1:16, NLT. This is what the Lord says: Why did you send messengers to Baal-zebub, the god of Ekron, to ask whether you will recover? Is there no God in Israel to answer your question?

201 Hab. 2:1-4, NLT. I will climb up to my watchtower and stand at my guardpost. There I will wait to see what the LORD says and how he will answer my complaint. Then the LORD said to me, "Write my answer plainly on tablets, so that a runner can carry

the correct message to others. This vision is for a future time. It describes the end, and it will be fulfilled. If it seems slow in coming, wait patiently, for it will surely take place. It will not be delayed.

202 Col. 2:2, AMPC. In Him all the treasures of [divine] wisdom (comprehensive insight into the ways and purposes of God) and [all the riches of spiritual] knowledge *and* enlightenment are stored up *and* lie hidden; Col. 2:2, MSB. The 1mandate of my ministry is for everyone's heart to be awakened to their true identity, 2intertwined in love's tapestry. This will launch you into a life of knowing the wealth of every 3conclusion and joint witness hidden within the mystery of God who fathered us and co-revealed us in Christ. ([1] The word, 1parakaleō, is often translated as comfort from para, a Preposition indicating close proximity; a thing proceeding from a sphere of influence, with a suggestion of union of place of residence; to have sprung from its author and giver; originating from, denoting the point from which an action originates; intimate connection; and kaleō, to surname, to identify by name, to call by name. [2] The phrase, 2sumbibatzō en agapē, means intertwined in love's tapestry; [3] and the word, σύνεσις 3sunesis, from suniemi, means joint seeing or understanding; a flowing together as of two streams - a seamless merging; a fusion of thought. It suggests the grasp and comprehension that happens from comparing and combining things.)

203 I Cor. 12:6-11, AMP. And there are [distinctive] ways of working [to accomplish things], but it is the same God who produces all things in all believers [inspiring, energizing, and empowering them]. But to each one is given the manifestation of the Spirit [the spiritual illumination and the enabling of the Holy Spirit] for the common good. To one is given through the [Holy] Spirit

[the power to speak] the message of wisdom, and to another [the power to express] the word of knowledge *and* understanding according to the same Spirit; to another [wonder-working] faith [is given] by the same [Holy] Spirit, and to another the [extraordinary] gifts of healings by the one Spirit; and to another the working of miracles, and to another prophecy [foretelling the future, speaking a new message from God to the people], and to another discernment of spirits [the ability to distinguish sound, godly doctrine from the deceptive doctrine of man-made religions and cults], to another *various* kinds of [unknown] tongues, and to another interpretation of tongues. All these things [the gifts, the achievements, the abilities, the empowering] are brought about by one and the same [Holy] Spirit, distributing to each one individually just as He chooses.

204 Isaiah 61:3, NLT. To all who mourn in Israel, he will give a crown of beauty for ashes, a joyous blessing instead of mourning, festive praise instead of despair. In their righteousness, they will be like great oaks that the Lord has planted for his own glory.

205 R. Laird Harris, Gleason L. Archer, and Bruce K. Waltke, eds., *Theological Wordbook of the Old Testament* (Chicago: Moody Press, 1980). *Shema (שָׁמַע)* – Entry #2443. Jesus reflects the Hebraic view in this verse. In Hebrew thought, "to obey" is not just about compliance—it's about attentive listening that leads to action. It's deeply relational. When God says, "Hear, O Israel…" (Deuteronomy 6:4), the word used is *Shema*, and it means: Hear + Understand + Internalize + Respond in trust and action. Obeying involves the heart, mind, and will—not just outward behavior. It reflects a love-based relationship, not a legalistic performance based one.

[206] John 14:21, TLB. See also John 14:20-21, in The Mirror Study Bible, MSB. I am in my Father, you are in me and I am in you. (The incarnation does not divide the Trinity; the incarnation celebrates the redeemed inclusion of humanity. Picture four circles with the one fitting into the other - The outer circle is the Father, then Jesus in the Father, then us in Jesus and the Holy Spirit in us. This spells inseparable, intimate oneness. Note that it is not our knowing that positions Jesus in the Father or us in them or the Spirit of Christ in us. Our knowing simply awakens us to the reality of our redeemed oneness. Gold does not become gold when it is discovered but it certainly becomes currency.) Verse 21 - Whoever 1resonates and 2treasures the 3completeness of my prophetic purpose cannot but fall in love with me and also find themselves to be fully participating in my Father's love and I will love this one and make myself distinctly known and real to each one individually. In this embrace of inseparable union, love rules. ([1] Intimacy is not the result of suspicious scrutiny but the inevitable fruit of trust. 1echō, to have; to hold; to resonate. [2] The word, 2tereō, means to treasure ; to safeguard. [3] The word 3entolē, which is often translated commandment or precept, or assignment, has two components, en, in and telos, from tellō, to set out for a definite point or goal; properly the point aimed at as a limit, that is, by implication, the conclusion of an act or state, the result; the ultimate or prophetic purpose. Strong's 5056.)

Chapter 16

[207] See Dallas Willard, Renewing the Christian Mind (New York: Harper One, 2016), 158–60, for his writings on gray matter and the soul to better understand the mind-brain relationship.

[208] Matt. 18:19-20, AMP. Again I say to you, that if two [a]believers on earth agree [that is, are of one mind, in harmony] about

anything that they ask [within the will of God], it will be done for them by My Father in heaven. For where two or three are gathered in My name [meeting together as My followers], I am there among them.

209 I John 4:18, NIRV. There is no fear in love. Instead, perfect love drives away fear.

210 John 10:10, AMP. The thief comes only in order to steal and kill and destroy. I came that they may have *and* enjoy life, and have it in abundance [to the full, till it overflows].

211 The thief comes only in order to steal and kill and destroy. I came that they may have and enjoy life, and have it in abundance [to the full, till it overflows].

212 Col. 4:2, NLT. Devote yourselves to prayer with an alert mind and a thankful heart; I Peter 5:8, MSG. Keep a cool head. Stay alert. The Devil is poised to pounce, and would like nothing better than to catch you napping. Keep your guard up. You're not the only ones plunged into these hard times. It's the same with Christians all over the world. So keep a firm grip on the faith. The suffering won't last forever. It won't be long before this generous God who has great plans for us in Christ—eternal and glorious plans they are!—will have you put together and on your feet for good. He gets the last word; yes, he does.

213 Dallas Willard, *Life Without Lack: Living in the Fullness of Psalm 23* (Nashville, TN: Thomas Nelson, 2018), 106.

214 Heb 4:15, NIRV. We have a high priest who can feel it when we are weak and hurting. Heb. 4:15, AMPC. For we do not have a High Priest who is unable to understand *and* sympathize and have a shared feeling with our weaknesses *and* infirmities.

215 Romans 8:26-27, J.B. Phillips. The Spirit of God not only maintains this hope within us, but helps us in our present limitations. For example, we do not know how to pray worthily as sons of God, but his Spirit within us is actually praying for us in those agonizing longings which never find words. And God who knows the heart's secrets understands, of course, the Spirit's intention as he prays for those who love God.

216 See John Piper, "He Helps Us in Our Weakness," a two-part series, *Desiring God*, https://www.desiringgod.org/messages/the-spirit-helps-us-in-our-weakness-part-1 and https://www.desiringgod.org/messages/the-spirit-helps-us-in-our-weakness-part-2. Be encouraged that God's work for you is not limited to what you can understand and express with words. God created the universe and all that is in it to display the riches of the glory of his grace. God gets glory because our hearts are made the theater for this divine activity, so that we know and experience God's gracious intercession for us and consciously give him thanks (Rom. 9:23).

217 Psalm 34:10, NKJV. But those who seek the Lord shall not lack any good thing; Psalm 34:10, Voice. But those intent on knowing the Eternal God will have everything they need.

218 John 1:14, AMP. The Word became a human being and lived here with us. We saw his true glory, the glory of the only Son of the Father. From him the complete gifts of undeserved grace and truth have come down to us.

219 Rev. 7:14, AMP. Salvation [belongs] to our God who is seated on the throne, and to the Lamb [our salvation is the Trinity's to give, and to God the Trinity we owe our deliverance]. The word salvation includes the idea of healing.

220 Isaiah 65:24, TLV. And it will come to pass that before they call, I will answer, and while they are still speaking, I will hear.

221 Psalm 141:8,9, Voice. My gaze is fixed upon You, Eternal One, my Lord; in You I find *safety and* protection. Do not *abandon me and* leave me defenseless. Protect me from the jaws of the trap my enemies have set for me and from the snares of those who work evil.

222 See Job 13:3-5, 13, ESV. Luke 4:35, ESV.

223 Psalm 43:2-4, NLT. Why must I wander around in grief, oppressed by my enemies? Send out your light and your truth; let them guide me. Let them lead me to your holy mountain, to the place where you live; John 1:14, NIV. The Word became flesh and made his dwelling among us. We have seen his glory, the glory of the one and only Son, who came from the Father, full of grace and truth.

224 Psalm 32:10, NLT. Unfailing love surrounds those who trust the Lord.

225 James 1:5, Voice. If you don't have all the wisdom needed *for this journey*, then all you have to do is ask God for it; and God will grant all that you need. He gives lavishly and never scolds you for asking.

226 John 5:19, 20, MSB. Jesus explained to them with utmost certainty that whatever they see the Son do, mirrors the Father - he does not act independent of his Father - the Son's gaze is fixed in order to accurately interpret and repeat what he sees his Father do. The one reveals the other without compromise or distraction. (The incarnation does not interrupt what the Word was from the beginning - face to face with God.) For the Father and the Son are best of friends. They have no secrets; the Father gladly lets his Son in on everything he does and will continue to show him works of most significant proportions, which will astound you. (The Father loves [phileo] the Son with fondness.)

227 John Mark Comer. *Practicing the Way: Be with Jesus, Become Like Him, Do as He Did* (Colorado Springs: Waterbrook, 2024), 4. Matt. 11:30, AMPC. My yoke is wholesome (useful, good—not harsh, hard, sharp, or pressing, but comfortable, gracious, and pleasant), and My burden is light and easy to be borne. 'Yoke' is a Hebrew idiom for a Rabbai's set of teachings, his way of reading Scripture, his take on how to thrive as a human being in God's good world. More resources are available at practicingtheway.org.

228 Phil. 2:13, MSG. Be energetic in your life of salvation, reverent and sensitive before God. That energy is *God's* energy, an energy deep within you, God himself willing and working at what will give him the most pleasure.

229 Ezek. 11:19-20, AMPC, And I will give them one heart [a new heart] and I will put a new spirit within them; and I will take the stony [unnaturally hardened] heart out of their flesh, and will give them a heart of flesh [sensitive and responsive to the touch of their God], that they may walk in My statutes and keep My ordinances, and do them. And they shall be My people, and I will be their God.

230 Prov. 18:20-21, NIV. From the fruit of their mouth a person's stomach is filled; with the harvest of their lips they are satisfied. The tongue has the power of life and death, and those who love it will eat its fruit.

231 Phil. 1:6, MSG. There has never been the slightest doubt in my mind that the God who started this great work in you would keep at it and bring it to a flourishing finish...

232 Jer. 32:41, NLT. And I will make an everlasting covenant with them: I will never stop doing good for them. I will put a desire in their hearts to worship me, and they will never leave me. I will

find joy doing good for them; John 15:11, AMP. I have told you these things so that My joy and delight may be in you, and that your joy may be made full and complete and overflowing.

233. Matt.9:12,13, AMPC. But when Jesus heard *this*, He said, "Those who are healthy have no need for a physician, but [only] those who are sick. Go and learn what this [Scripture] means: 'I desire compassion [for those in distress], and not [animal] sacrifice,' for I did not come to call [to repentance] the [self-proclaimed] righteous [who see no need to change], but sinners [those who recognize their sin and actively seek forgiveness].

234. Psalm 91:15, ESV. When he calls to Me I will answer him; I will be with him in trouble; I will rescue him and honor him. Psalm 118:5, ESV. Out of my distress I called on the Lord; the Lord answered me and set me free.

235. Isaiah 65:24, TLB. I will answer them before they even call to me. While they are still talking to me about their needs I will go ahead and answer their prayers.

236. Jeremiah 33:2-3, ESV. Thus says the Lord who made the earth, the Lord who formed it to establish it – the Lord is his name. Call to me and I will answer you, and tell you great and hidden things that you have not known.

237. Luke 9:23, The MSG. Jesus told them what they could expect for themselves: "Anyone who intends to come with me has to let me lead. You're not in the driver's seat – I am. Don't run from suffering; embrace it. Follow me and I'll show you how."

Chapter 17

238. Apraxia is a speech problem caused by the brain's inability to deliver correct movement instructions to the tongue, mouth,

and jaw. It's a common challenge among individuals with Down syndrome.

239 Psalm 121:3, ESV. He who keeps you will not slumber. See also Psalm 103.

240 Job 33:15, NLT. He speaks in dreams, in visions of the night, when deep sleep falls on people as they lie in their beds.

241 Hebrews 5:14, MSB. This is the nourishment of the mature. They are those who have their faculties of perception trained as by gymnastic precision to distinguish the relevant from the irrelevant.

Chapter 18

242 Psalm 31:9,10,14,15, NIV. Be merciful to me, Lord, for I am in distress, my eyes grow weak with sorrow, my soul and body with grief. My life is consumed by anguish and my years by groaning; my strength fails because of my affliction, and my bones grow weak. But I trust in you, Lord; I say, "You are my God. My times are in your hand."

243 I Cor. 12:7, ESV. To each is given the manifestation of the Spirit for the common good.

Chapter 19

244 Bessel A. Van der Kolk, *The Body Keeps the Score: Brain, Mind, and Body in the Healing of Trauma* (New York: Viking Press, Penguin Random House, 2014), 17.

245 A. W. Tozer, *Knowledge of the Holy* (New York: Harper Collins, 1961), 1.

246 Ruth Burrows, *Essence of Prayer* (Hidden Springs, 2006), 1.

247 John 5:17, 19-20 NLT. Jesus replied, "My Father is always working, and so am I... I tell you the truth, the Son can do nothing by himself. He does only what he sees the Father doing. Whatever the Father does, the Son also does. For the Father loves the Son and shows him everything he is doing. In fact, the Father will show him how to do even greater works than healing this man. Then you will truly be astonished.

248 Ruth Burrows, *Ibid.*, 2.

249 2 Cor 3:18, ESV. And we all, with unveiled face, beholding the glory of the Lord, are being transformed into the same image from one degree of glory to another. For this comes from the Lord who is the Spirit.

250 Micah 7:9, TLB. God will bring me out of my darkness into the light, and I will see his goodness.

251 Ex. 20:6, NLT. But I lavish unfailing love for a thousand generations on those who love me and obey my commands.

252 Hebrews 12:13, MSB. Get rid of all obstacles that could possibly cause you to stumble and sprain an ankle. Don't let recurrent injury force you out of the race. Recover and carry on running. Don't allow old legalistic mind-sets to trip you up again.

253 For a step-by-step guide of this natural calming/acute focus tool used by special ops teams in high-threat situations, go to https://www.pamvredevelt.com/free-resources

254 Isaiah 26:3, NLT. You will keep in perfect peace all who trust in you, all whose thoughts are fixed on you!

255 Psalm 23:6, NLT. Surely your goodness and unfailing love will pursue me all the days of my life, and I will live in the house of the Lord forever.

256 Romans 8:1, NLT. So now there is no condemnation for those who belong to Christ Jesus.

257 Hebrews 10:19-23, ERV. And so, brothers and sisters, we are completely free to enter the Most Holy Place (the spiritual place God lives and is worshiped). We can do this without fear because of the blood sacrifice of Jesus. We enter through a new way that Jesus opened for us. It is a living way that leads through the curtain—Christ's body…Sprinkled with the blood of Christ, our hearts have been made free from a guilty conscience, and our bodies have been washed with pure water. So come near to God with a sincere heart, full of confidence because of our faith in Christ. We must hold on to the hope we have, never hesitating to tell people about it. We can trust God to do what he promised.

258 Isaiah 53:3-5, ESV. He was despised and rejected by men, a man of sorrows and acquainted with grief; Surely he has borne our griefs and carried our sorrows…upon him was the chastisement that brought us peace, and with his wounds we are healed.

259 Gen 16:13, Voice. As a result of this encounter, Hagar decided to give the Eternal One who had spoken to her a special name because He had seen her in her misery. Hagar: I'm going to call You the God of Seeing because in this place I have seen the One who watches over me; AMPC. So, Hagar called the name of the Lord Who spoke to her, You are a God of seeing, for she said, Have I not even here in the wilderness looked upon Him Who sees me and lived? Or have I here also seen the future purposes or designs of Him Who sees me?

260 Isaiah 45:3, TLB. And I will give you treasures hidden in the darkness, secret riches; and you will know that I am doing this—I, the Lord, the God of Israel, the one who calls you by your name.

261 Isaiah 49:15-16, EHV. Can a woman forget her nursing child and not show mercy to the son from her womb? Even if these women could forget, I will never forget you. Look, I have inscribed you on the palms of my hands. Your walls are never out of my sight.

262 John 10:29, MSG. My sheep recognize my voice. I know them, and they follow me. I give them real and eternal life. They are protected from the Destroyer for good. No one can steal them from out of my hand. The Father who put them under my care is so much greater than the Destroyer and Thief. No one could ever get them away from him. I and the Father are one heart and mind.

263 Rom. 8:38,39, NLT. And I am convinced that nothing can ever separate us from God's love. Neither death nor life, neither angels nor demons, neither our fears for today nor our worries about tomorrow—not even the powers of hell can separate us from God's love. No power in the sky above or in the earth below—indeed, nothing in all creation will ever be able to separate us from the love of God that is revealed in Christ Jesus our Lord.

264 Psalm 23:6, AMP. Surely goodness and mercy and unfailing love shall follow me all the days of my life, And I shall dwell forever [throughout all my days] in the house *and* in the presence of the Lord.

265 2 Chron. 16:9, NLT.

266 Is. 61:1-3, TLB. The Spirit of the Lord God is upon me, because the Lord has anointed me to bring good news to the suffering and afflicted. He has sent me to comfort the brokenhearted, to announce liberty to captives, and to open the eyes of the blind. He has sent me to tell those who mourn that the time of God's favor to them has come, and the day of his wrath to their enemies.

To all who mourn…he will give: beauty for ashes; joy instead of mourning; praise instead of heaviness. For God has planted them like strong and graceful oaks for his own glory.

267. Romans 14:17, NLT. For the Kingdom of God is…living a life of goodness and peace and joy in the Holy Spirit.

268. James 1:17, Voice. Every good gift bestowed, every perfect gift received comes to us from above, courtesy of the Father of lights. He *is consistent*. He won't change His mind or play tricks in the shadows.

269. Jeremiah 31:33, MSG. I will put my law within them—write it on their hearts!—and be their God. And they will be my people. They will no longer go around setting up schools to teach each other about God. They'll know me firsthand, the dull and the bright, the smart and the slow. I'll wipe the slate clean for each of them. I'll forget they ever sinned!" God's Decree.

Chapter 20

270. Psalm 55:22, AMP. Cast your burden on the LORD release it and He will sustain *and* uphold you; He will never allow the righteous to be shaken (slip, fall, fail).

271. John 16:27, AMP. "The Father Himself [tenderly] loves you, because you have loved Me and have believed that I came from the Father"

272. John 14:21, AMP. "The person who has My commandments and keeps them is the one who really loves Me; and whoever really loves Me will be loved by My Father, and I will love him and reveal Myself to him I will make Myself real to him."

273. Gen. 16:13, AMPC. Then she called the name of the Lord who spoke to her, "You are God Who Sees"; for she said, "Have I not

even here in the wilderness remained alive after seeing Him who sees me with understanding and compassion?"

274 I John 3:1, NIV. See what great love the Father has lavished on us, that we should be called children of God! And that is what we are!

275 Galatians 4:5-7, The MSG. Thus, we have been set free to experience our rightful heritage. You can tell for sure that you are now fully adopted as his own children because God sent the Spirit of his Son into our lives crying out, "Papa! Father!" Doesn't that privilege of intimate conversation with God make it plain that you are not a slave, but a child? And if you are a child, you're also an heir, with complete access to the inheritance.

276 Gretchen Schmelzer, "The Healing Power of Poetry," *Journey Through Trauma* blog, April 21, 2024, from *Journey Through Trauma: A Trail Guide Through the 5-Phase Cycle of Healing Repeated Trauma* (New York: Avery, 2018).

277 James Nestor, Breath: *The New Science of a Lost Art* (New York: Riverhead Books, 2020), 221. Coherent Breathing—Inhale softly for 5 to 6 seconds filling the lungs while extending the belly, then slowly exhale 5 to 6 seconds. Repeat ten or more times. This tool brings the heart, lungs and circulation into a state of coherence, where body systems are working at peak efficiency. For coherent breathing and related research, see this book.

278 Hebrew 11:6, NLT. And it is impossible to please God without faith. Anyone who wants to come to him must believe that God exists and that he rewards those who sincerely seek him.

279 I Peter 1:2, AMPC. To you who were chosen and foreknown by God the Father and consecrated (sanctified, made holy) by the Spirit to be obedient to Jesus Christ (the Messiah) and to be sprinkled with His blood: May grace (spiritual blessing) and

peace be given you in increasing abundance that spiritual peace to be realized in and through Christ, freedom from fears, agitating passions, and moral conflicts.

280 I Peter 2:24, NKJV.

281 John 14:2, MSB. Jesus said, 'What makes my Father's house home, is your place in it. If this was not the ultimate conclusion of my mission, why would I even bother to do what I am about to do if it was not to prepare a place for you? I have come to persuade you of a place of seamless oneness where you belong.'

282 James 4:8, NLT.

Chapter 21

283 Martha Graham created a dance technique that became the first significant alternative to classical ballet. Graham was the first creator of modern dance to devise a truly universal dance technique out of the movements she developed in her choreography. Her dance language was intended to express shared human emotions and experiences, rather than merely provide decorative displays of graceful movements. The Martha Graham School of Contemporary Dance has the distinction of being the longest continuously operating school of dance in the United States. See Martha Graham Center of Contemporary Dance, "About Martha Graham," *Martha Graham Dance Company*, accessed Aug 30, 2024, https://marthagraham.org/martha-graham/.

284 I'm quoting Ruth Haley Barton with a minor adjustment who insightfully said, "The best gift you can give the people you lead is your transforming self." https://transformingcenter.org/strengthening-the-soul-of-your-leadership-podcast/

285 I Peter 5:6-7, AMP. Therefore, humble yourselves under the mighty hand of God [set aside self-righteous pride], so that He may exalt you at the appropriate time, casting all your cares (all your anxieties, all your worries, and all your concerns, once and for all) on Him, for He cares about you with deepest affection, and watches over you very carefully.

286 I Peter 5:6-7, AMP. Therefore, humble yourselves under the mighty hand of God [set aside self-righteous pride], so that He may exalt you at the appropriate time, casting all your cares (all your anxieties, all your worries, and all your concerns, once and for all) on Him, for He cares about you with deepest affection, and watches over you very carefully.

287 Psalm 130:5-7, The MSG. I pray to God—my life a prayer—and wait for what he'll say and do. My life is on the line before God, my Lord, waiting and watching till morning, waiting and watching till morning… wait and watch for God—with God's arrival comes love, with God's arrival comes generous redemption.

288 Hebrews 4:1, 5-16, NIV. For we do not have a high priest who is unable to empathize with our weaknesses, but we have one who has been tempted in every way, just as we are—yet he did not sin. 16 Let us then approach God's throne of grace with confidence, so that we may receive mercy and find grace to help us in our time of need.

289 Eph. 4:23, NLT. Instead, let the Spirit renew your thoughts and attitudes.

290 Jenny Donelly, is an author, speaker, and founder of Her Voice Movement HVMT. She oversees prayer hubs where women gather once a month in homes across the country to pray for the

turning of our nation back to God and positive change in every sphere of culture.

291 Matt. 13:11-12, NLT. Jesus replied, "You are permitted to understand the secrets of the Kingdom of Heaven, but others are not. To those who listen to my teaching, more understanding will be given, and they will have an abundance of knowledge.; I Cor 2:9-11, NLT. That is what the Scriptures mean when they say, "No eye has seen, no ear has heard, and no mind has imagined what God has prepared for those who love him." But it was to us that God revealed these things by his Spirit. For his Spirit searches out everything and shows us God's deep secrets.

292 Is 45:3, NLT. And I will give you treasures hidden in the darkness— secret riches. I will do this so you may know that I am the Lord, the God of Israel, the one who calls you by name.

293 Prov. 8:14, 17-21, 34-35 AMP. Counsel is mine and sound wisdom; I am understanding, power *and* strength are mine... I love those who love me; And those who seek me early *and* diligently will find me. Riches and honor are with me, Enduring wealth and righteousness (right standing with God). My fruit is better than gold, even pure gold, and my yield is better than choicest silver. I, [Wisdom, continuously] walk in the way of righteousness, In the midst of the paths of justice, That I may cause those who love me to inherit wealth *and* true riches, and that I may fill their treasuries… Blessed [happy, prosperous, to be admired] is the man who listens to me, watching daily at my gates, waiting at my doorposts. For whoever finds me (Wisdom) finds life and obtains favor *and* grace from the Lord.

294 Eph. 3:16, 18, 20, AMP. May He grant you out of the riches of His glory, to be strengthened *and* spiritually energized with power through His Spirit in your inner self, [indwelling your innermost

being and personality], 17 so that Christ may dwell in your hearts through your faith... and [that you may come] to know [practically, through personal experience] the love of Christ which far surpasses [mere] knowledge [without experience], that you may be filled up [throughout your being] to all the fullness of God [so that you may have the richest experience of God's presence in your lives, completely filled and flooded with God Himself]... who is able to [carry out His purpose and] do superabundantly more than all that we dare ask or think [infinitely beyond our greatest prayers, hopes, or dreams], according to His power that is at work within us.

295 Isaiah 61:3, TLB. To all who mourn he will give: beauty for ashes; joy instead of mourning; praise instead of heaviness. For God has planted them like strong and graceful oaks for his own glory.

296 Randy Alcorn, *The Promise of the New Earth: Reflections on Our Eternal Home* (Sandy, OR: Eternal Perspectives Ministries, 2022). See also his devotional, *50 Days of Heaven: Reflections That Bring Eternity to Light*, based on his full-length book *Heaven*, which I read several times after Nathan relocated to Heaven. A complete list of Alcorn's books can be found at epm.org/books.

297 Credit and thanks to my friend Paul Young for coining the term 'redeeming genius.' Paul is the best-selling author of *The Shack: Where Tragedy Confronts Eternity* (Ventura, CA: Windblown Media, 2007).

298 See further details and examples in 2 Cor 3:17, Joel 2:28,29 and Acts 2:17,18; Isaiah 61 and Luke 4:14-20; Ezekial 3:12, Ezekial 37, Ezekial 43:4-6, 2 Peter 1:21, John 3:8, Acts 3:39.

299 2 Cor. 4:6-10, 16-18, ICB. God once said, "Let the light shine out of the darkness!" And this is the same God who made his light shine in our hearts. He gave us light by letting us know the glory of God that is in the face of Christ. We have this treasure from God. But we are only like clay jars that hold the treasure. This shows that this great power is from God, not from us. We have troubles all around us, but we are not defeated. We do not know what to do, but we do not give up. We are persecuted, but God does not leave us. We are hurt sometimes, but we are not destroyed. 10 We carry the death of Jesus in our own bodies, so that the life of Jesus can also be seen in our bodies. So, we do not give up. Our physical body is becoming older and weaker, but our spirit inside us is made new every day. We have small troubles for a while now, but they are helping us gain an eternal glory. That glory is much greater than the troubles. So, we set our eyes not on what we see but on what we cannot see. What we see will last only a short time. But what we cannot see will last forever.

Acknowledgements

This book is the work of many hearts and hands. It could not have come to life without the unwavering love, support, and encouragement of my husband, John, and our adult children, Jessie and Benjamin.

To those referenced in the endnotes—my heartfelt gratitude. Dallas Willard, John Mark Comer, Andy Crouch, Jamie Winship, John Ortberg, Tish Harrison Warren, and others—your wisdom has stretched, challenged, and inspired me over the years to think deeply, explore courageously, question honestly, pray continually—and then begin the cycle all over again.

To my wise companions who read early drafts and offered thoughtful feedback—Chuck Walker, Charles Kind, Mary Kruze, Jesse Vance, Craig Ancel, Marilyn Williams, Gail Gunstone, and Kathie Kyono—your insights helped shape this manuscript into a more beautiful gift for the reader who chooses to receive it.

To the talented creatives who brought visual beauty to this work—Maddy Ferrara, Karen Bressel, and Sarah Rodrigues—your artistry lifted the heart and message of *Mending Miracles* to another level.

To my editor, Judith, and amazing pre-reading team—Joy Marsh, Donna Chaney, Debbie Woods, and Carla Miller—thank you for your countless hours, keen eyes, and the grace with which you helped refine each line and gently erase my mistakes.

And finally, my heartfelt gratitude to JJ Hebert, for supporting this message, and to Monica Kelly, marketing and technology wizard extraordinaire, whose strategic insight and hands-on implementation are helping get Mending Miracles to those who eagerly long for hope and healing.

Each of you is a treasured gift.

BEST-SELLING POPULAR RESOURCES BY PAM VREDEVELT

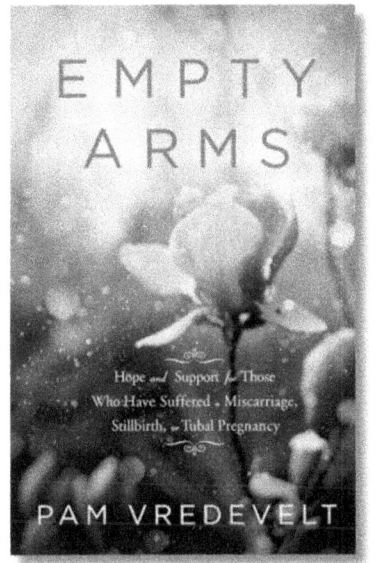

They are the most dreaded words an expectant mother can hear.

As joy and anticipation dissolve into confusion and grief, painful questions refuse to go away:

Why me?
What did I do wrong?
Does God care?
Now what?

With the warmth and compassion of a seasoned professional counselor and a Christian woman who has suffered miscarriage herself, Pam Vredevelt offers sound neuroscience-backed answers, timeless wisdom, and Biblical reassurance to the woman longing to maintain faith and proactively work with this heartbreaking situation. Pam's accompanying journal guides you with simple daily action steps to gently release grief and receive God's healing love.

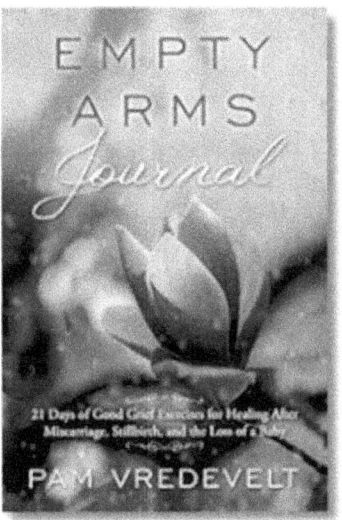

 BOOK ←

JOURNAL →

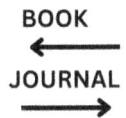 

SCAN THE QR CODE TO WATCH HEALING AFTER PREGNANCY LOSS

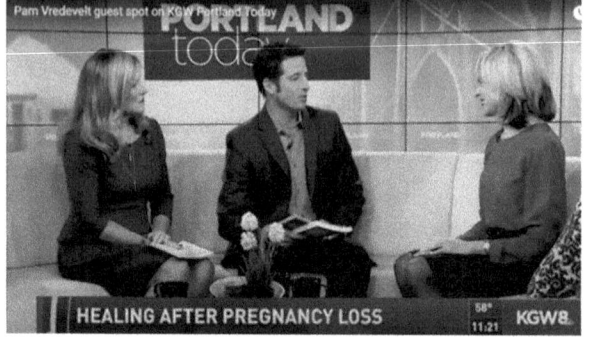

Have you suffered the loss of your baby or child?

Do sorrow, guilt, grief and anger threaten to sweep you away?

Do you feel like you're grieving alone and that no one truly understands what you're going through?

 I INVITE YOU TO EXCHANGE THE HOLLOW EMPTINESS OF GRIEF FOR GOD'S HEALING ENCOUNTERS AND WHOLENESS.

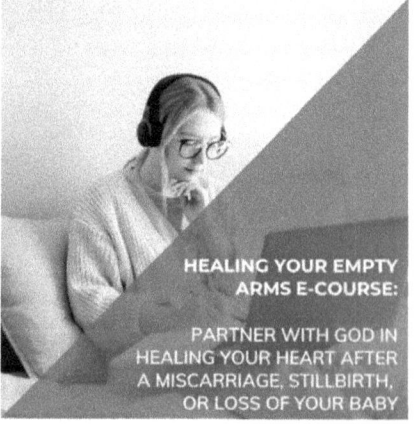

HEALING YOUR EMPTY ARMS E-COURSE:

PARTNER WITH GOD IN HEALING YOUR HEART AFTER A MISCARRIAGE, STILLBIRTH, OR LOSS OF YOUR BABY

In HEALING YOUR EMPTY ARMS, we will travel a healing path together, step-by-step through your grief. You'll learn how to receive God's grace and safely release the emotions that are often blocked and buried in a shattered heart. You'll be equipped with neuroscience and Scripture-based practical tools to process your loss in ways that promote healing, peace, and meaning.

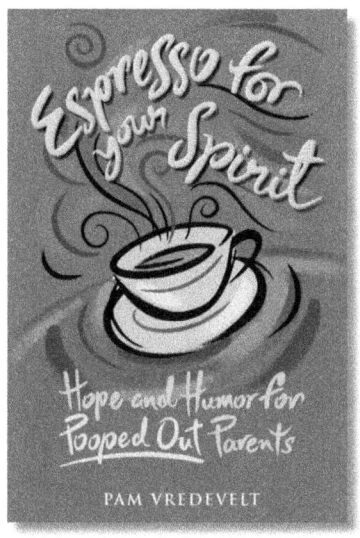

HOPE AND HUMOR FOR POOPED OUT PARENTS

It's no secret that parenting is overwhelming and often exhausting. Nothing will ever change the daunting struggles parents face and the tears often shed. The daily grind of dirty diapers, soccer games, fund-raisers, and bloody knees leaves parents needing a resource that will lift their spirits, charge their batteries, and refocus them on the source of their true strength. In engaging, read-to-your-kids humorous quips, and poignant vignettes.

Bestselling author Pam Vredevelt serves up cup after cup of energizing espresso to encourage worn-out parents and make the whole family laugh.

YOUR DAILY 5-MINUTE TRANSFORMATION TOOL

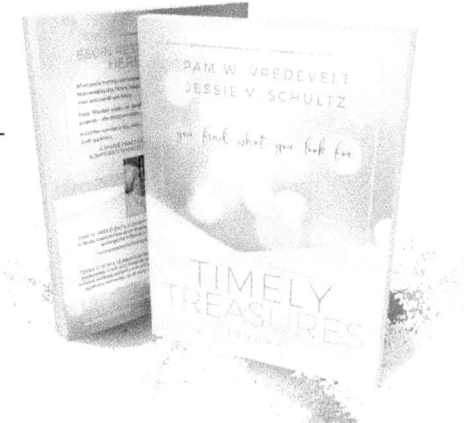

Scan to Learn More

www.ingramcontent.com/pod-product-compliance
Lightning Source LLC
Chambersburg PA
CBHW061214070526
44584CB00029B/3829